THE VACCINATION CONTROVERSY

THE
VACCINATION
CONTROVERSY

*The rise, reign and fall of
compulsory vaccination for smallpox*

Stanley Williamson

Liverpool University Press

First published 2007 by
Liverpool University Press
4 Cambridge Street
Liverpool L69 7ZU

British Library Cataloguing-in-Publication data
A British Library CIP record is available

ISBN 978-1-84631-086-7 cased
978-1-84631-087-4 limp

Typeset by XL Publishing Services, Tiverton
Printed and bound in the European Union by Bell and Bain Ltd, Glasgow

For

Bettie and Elisabeth

In England in the nineteenth century vaccination was the subject of the greatest controversy in the history of medicine. The literature on the subject is enormous...

C. W. Dixon, *Smallpox*, 1962

Every individual who has undergone Vaccine inoculation correctly is for ever rescued from contagion of the Small Pox.

Edward Jenner, 1803

An Act further to extend and make compulsory the Practice of Vaccination.

16 and 17, Vict., c.100, 1853

We abhor the rite. We detest it as an imposture. We dread it as a danger. We refute it on any terms. We encourage, we justify, we insist on the duty of rejection.

William White, *The Story of a Great Delusion*, 1885

... care must be taken to discriminate between what can be done by legislation for the people and what can only be accomplished by themselves individually and swayed by the slow progress of opinion.

William Farr, 1843

CONTENTS

ACKNOWLEDGEMENTS

For assisting my research and granting me permission to quote from their own work I gratefully acknowledge my indebtedness to: the John Rylands Library; the Library of the Manchester Medical Society; the University Library of Manchester; the Library of the Royal College of Physicians; Leicestershire Record Office; Manchester Central Library; Cheshire Library; Norwich Library; Sir Cyril A. Clarke FRCP FRS; Professor Roy Macleod; Dr M. L. Millard; Dr R. Houlton; Joan Egan; Mrs J. C. Sen.

I must also offer my sincere thanks to my mentor, Ian Moffitt, and to my daughter, Elisabeth Sullivan, for the many hours they devoted to rescuing a computer illiterate from the consequences of his own blunders, and above all to Mildred Marney whose patience and encouragement throughout what proved to be an exceptionally long haul have contributed far more to the completed work than simply the processing of the words.

PART I

The Road to Compulsion

CHAPTER 1

THE BYZANTINE OPERATION

During the early part of 1716 a caravan of coaches and wagons, bearing an English family and their numerous retinue, rumbled across Europe towards Constantinople. The journey could have been more easily and cheaply made by sea, but Edward Wortley Montagu, newly appointed Ambassador Extraordinary to the Sublime Porte, had decided that the special mission he was entrusted with might stand a greater chance of success if he called in at Vienna on the way.

The Ottoman Empire at that time still thrust deep into south-east Europe. Attempts by the Turks to push the frontier even further westward had been foiled in 1683, when their assault on Vienna was repulsed. But the two imperialisms, Turkish and Austro-Hungarian, still faced each other with mutual antipathy, which in 1716 seemed likely to break out again into open hostility. For complex reasons the British government was anxious that the Austrians should not be caught up in a war in eastern Europe, and the new ambassador's task was to try to head them off and reach some form of settlement with the Turks.

Wortley Montagu was accompanied by his wife, Lady Mary, and their three-year-old son, Edward junior. Lady Mary enjoyed travelling and was said to be 'charmed with thoughts of going into the East', which was just as well. The initial appointment was for a period of five years, but for all they knew they might be going into a long and possibly permanent exile.

The ambassador's negotiations in Vienna were largely unprofitable and after a brief stay the party set out towards the end of March 1717 on the next stage of their journey. This took them as far as Adrianople (now Edirne), at that time the capital of the Turkish empire, to which the Sultan usually retired in order to escape the summer heat of Constantinople. From the time of their entry into Turkey, Lady Mary embarked with enthusiasm on the course known to later generations as 'going native'. She learned Turkish. She took to dressing Turkish style and had her portrait painted in Turkish costume. She became friendly with Turkish ladies of standing and seized every opportunity of being admitted to the intimacy of the harem, coming to the unexpected conclusion that Turkish women led freer and more pleasurable lives than did English women. She visited the women's baths, but tactfully declined the pressing invitations of her hostesses to join them in their communal nudity. All this and much more she described in carefully composed letters to her friends in England, gently and rather unfairly mocking their ignorance of life in a faraway land which most of them would never be able to see for themselves.

Among her correspondence one letter stands out and has been much quoted for its importance in the history of preventive medicine. It was addressed from Adrianople to her friend Sarah Chiswell, who had chosen not to accompany her on the journey.

> The small-pox, so fatal, and so general among us, is here entirely harmless by the invention of *ingrafting*, which is the name they give it. There is a set of old women who make it their business to perform the operation every autumn, in the month of September, when the great heat is abated. People send to one another to know if any of their family has a mind to have the small pox: they make parties for this purpose, and when they are met (commonly fifteen or sixteen together) the old woman comes with a nut-shell full of the best sort of small-pox, and asks what veins you please to have opened. She immediately rips open that you offer her with a large needle (which gives you no more pain than a common scratch), and puts into the vein as much venom as can lie on the head of her needle, and after binds up the little wound with a hollow bit of shell; and in this manner opens four or five veins [...] The children or young patients play together all the rest of the day, and are in perfect health to the eighth. Then the fever begins to seize them, and they keep to their beds two days, very seldom three. They have very rarely above twenty or thirty [pocks] in their faces, which never mark; and in eight days time they are as well as before their illness... every year thousands undergo this operation, and the French ambassador says pleasantly, that they take the small-pox here by way of diversion, as they take the waters in other countries.[1]

The crucial fact, omitted from Lady Mary's letter because Sarah Chiswell would not have needed reminding of it, was that smallpox was one of the eruptive diseases, like measles, whose peculiarity, inexplicable at the time, was that a victim lucky enough to survive an attack would almost certainly never suffer another. The point of the Byzantine operation was to have the disease in the attenuated form of 'ingrafting', or inoculation, and hence be protected thereafter from the 'natural' disease. To a strong-minded mother with a young child's welfare at heart the assurance that the procedure appeared to offer was a compelling attraction, especially in view of its alleged safety. 'There is no example of any one that has died in it; and you may believe I am very well satisfied of the safety of the experiment, since I intend to try it on my dear little son.'

This was a momentous step and at first sight seems unlikely to have been envisaged without some consultation with the child's father, but if her choice of words is to be taken at face value the initiative must have lain with Lady Mary, and would have been all of a piece with the course of their marriage, then in its fifth year. Lady Mary's father, Lord Dorchester (later the Earl of Kingston), had chosen as her prospective husband the Honourable Clatworthy Skeffington, about whom little seems to be known except that he would not have been Lady Mary's choice, as she demonstrated by eloping with Wortley Montagu, after some typical procrastination on his part, and marrying him in 1712. This was an inauspicious entry into marriage, not helped by her father's predictable rage and the behaviour of her cold fish of a husband, who was eleven years older than herself.

Edward junior, their first child, was born in May 1713 and was, or so his mother seems to have feared, rather frail, giving her cause for much anxiety. Above all, like most parents at that time, she lived with the ever-present dread of smallpox. Throughout the eighteenth century, in London alone, the annual total of deaths from the disease rarely fell below 500, and frequently rose above 3,000. Among the 1,614 victims in 1713, a year of severe epidemic, was Lady Mary's brother, a young man of twenty-one who died leaving a wife and two children. Her passionate grief for his loss was made even more unbearable by her fears for her husband, at the mercy of the disease in the capital while she and their son were living temporarily in the comparative safety of the countryside near York.

I fright myself with imaginary horrors and shall always be fancying dangers while you are out of my sight [...] there wants but little of my being afraid of the small-pox for you, so unreasonable are my fears which however proceed from my unlimited love [...] since the loss of my poor unhappy brother I dread every evil.

Two years later, in December 1715, the evil she so much feared struck, but the victim was herself. By this time she was back in London, able to be attended by the best doctors, for whom she acquired a lasting contempt on account of their supposed incompetence. The disease, although sparing her life, bequeathed her the familiar legacy of disfigurement. Previously noted for her beauty, she was, according to contemporary accounts, left with no eyelashes (she was fortunate not to have lost her sight) and with a superabundance of pockmarks on her face. This misfortune, following the far greater tragedy of her brother's death, is sufficient to explain her readiness to have the experiment of 'ingrafting' tried on her young son.

Although she took the decision while in Adrianople she delayed making preparations for the operation until they were all settled in Pera, the fashionable quarter of Constantinople overlooking the Golden Horn, where the foreign diplomats and business community were mostly to be found. The final step was taken in March 1717 while Edward was away on a lengthy visit to Belgrade, where he received news of the operation in a letter written five days afterwards: 'The boy was ingrafted last Tuesday and is at this time singing and playing, and very impatient for his supper. I pray God my next may give as good an account of him...' The second bulletin reported him as being well and out of danger, though his father apparently remained true to form. 'Your son is very well,' Lady Mary wrote in a third letter, adding, 'I cannot forbear telling you so, though you do not so much as ask after him.'

The engrafting of young Edward proved in reality a less happy-go-lucky affair than the festive occasion implied by Lady Mary's letter to Sarah Chiswell. She herself left no known description but an account was later published by a man who was called upon to play an unexpected part in it. Charles Maitland was a Scottish surgeon whom Wortley Montagu had invited to take charge of the family's health during the long and potentially fraught journey to Constantinople. He claimed in his narrative to have 'long heard of the famous practice of transplanting or raising the small-pox by inoculation'. He, and indeed Lady Mary, had presumably read or at least heard of the accounts published two or three years earlier in the *Philosophical Transactions* of the Royal Society. As the author of one of them, Emanuel Timoni, was employed by Wortley Montagu as physician to the family while they were in Constantinople, Lady Mary would almost certainly have taken his advice into account in coming to her crucial decision.[2] It was to Maitland, however, that she entrusted the handling of the business.

'She first of all order'd me to find a fit subject [i.e. a smallpox patient] to take the matter from and then sent for an old Greek woman who had practis'd this way a great many years. After a good deal of trouble I found a proper subject....'[3] There was no jolly party of like-minded parents and other candidates for the needle: this was to be a private venture, at least until the outcome was known, and in view of the turn taken by events this arrangement was a wise one. Allowing for Maitland's understandable desire to show his own contribution in the best light the operation seems to have been deplorably bungled:

> the good woman went to work: but so awkwardly by the shaking of her hand and put the child to so much torture by her blunt and rusty needle, that I pitied his cries, who had ever been of such spirit and courage that hardly any thing of pain could make him cry before; and therefore I inoculated the other arm with my own instrument, and with so little pain to him that he did not in the least complain of it.

The aftermath of the operation was less traumatic. The disease followed a fairly mild course, as predicted, allowing Lady Mary to send the favourable reports to her husband. How might she, in the circumstances, have faced breaking the news of a less favourable outcome?

A curious sidelight on the episode was revealed several years later, when young Edward, indulging in one of his favourite pastimes, absconded from school. Rather as though he were a runaway slave an advertisement was issued offering twenty pounds reward 'and reasonable charges' for his recapture. He had, it was stated, 'two marks by which he is easily known – viz. on the back of each arm, about two inches above the wrist, a small rounded scar, less than a silver penny, like a large mark of the small-pox'. These were presumably the result of his operation. Maitland's account had stressed the absence of marks when the wounds caused by the inoculation had healed.

By 1718 Wortley Montagu was perceived as having made an unacceptable hash of his mission, although he vehemently denied it; at all events, the government peremptorily summoned him home and sent out a replacement. The family, which now included a baby daughter, returned to London and set about the task of rebuilding their lives after their brief adventure in the capital of the Ottoman Empire.

CHAPTER 2

THE SMALL POCKES

Opening their account of the campaign conducted by the World Health Organization that in 1979 finally extinguished, or, as their forerunners might have said, 'extirpated' smallpox from the earth, the authors remark: 'The majority of people – including the majority of physicians – now living have never seen a case of this once dreaded disease'. In the years since that number will have declined even further, and it therefore seems desirable to recall something of the history and characteristics of the disease which once inspired so much dread.

The early history of smallpox is one of the areas in which the uninstructed traveller trying to find his way is most likely to lose it. Accounts are littered with signposts indicating paths that 'may' lead in the right direction, or destinations that 'could have been' the one being sought. Dates hazarded for remote events, such as the emergence of smallpox as a disease of animals, or its transference to human beings, may vary by several thousand years. 'Plagues' or 'pestilences' referred to could have been examples of any one of a number of diseases incorporating some sort of rash, a difficulty complicated over the centuries by what one authority describes as 'the uncertainties of translation'. The most common candidates for confusion include smallpox, measles, chickenpox, scarlet fever and erysipelas, any one of which the puzzled pathfinder may conclude is interchangeable with any of the others. Students of etymology may be interested in the attempt of Creighton, the great historian of epidemics, to unravel some of the more recondite examples.[1]

The most commonly accepted sequence of events is that smallpox emerged as a disease of some species of animal in Africa in prehistoric times, was somehow transferred to human beings and eventually found a route to the Far East. Creighton disposed of this earlier migration somewhat summarily: 'the evidence of the antiquity of smallpox in China and India may be accepted and for the rest left out of account'.

This dismissive pronouncement deprives us of colourful accounts of gods and goddesses of plague and smallpox, of the introduction some two thousand years ago of the Chinese method of inoculation by way of the nose, and of evidence from other sources pre-dating its arrival in the Orient of the possible existence of smallpox in Egypt in the second millennium BC, as suggested by the condition of a number of mummies, including that of Rameses V, who may have been a victim.

There is a consensus, otherwise rare, among historians that the classical civilizations of Greece and Rome were spared epidemics or even isolated examples of smallpox, a conclusion resting on the absence of any reference to it, either by name or by recognizable symptoms, in the documents of the period. Numerous attempts have been made to interpret as smallpox the plague or pestilence that ravaged Athens in 434 BC, as described by Thucydides, who lived through it, but they have usually broken down over some point of importance, with an epidemic of measles or typhus suggested as possible alternatives.

The early incursion of smallpox into Europe is marked by alleged sightings for which reliable confirmation is mostly lacking. Gregory of Tours describes something resembling smallpox in AD 580, though it may have been plague. The disease is said to have appeared among the Abyssinian army that besieged Mecca in 569 or 571; the tradition rests on word of mouth only but the normally sceptical Creighton surprisingly comments that it 'need not on that account be set aside as worthless'. Then there is St Nicaise, Bishop of Rheims, who, before his martyrdom at the hands of marauding Huns in 406 (he miraculously, but only temporarily, survived the severance and replacement of his head), had allegedly recovered from an attack of smallpox and subsequently became the patron saint of victims of the disease.

It was held at one time that smallpox was probably brought to western Europe by crusaders returning from the Holy Land, but this assumption lacked reliable confirmation. It was succeeded by evidence that placed the transition several centuries earlier, with the sudden transformation of Arabia from the relative obscurity of a 'backward' country of whose existence, as Fisher put it, 'no European statesman had occasion to remember',[2] into a great and expanding military power. Among the forces that in the seventh and eighth centuries brought large parts of Asia, North Africa and southern Europe under Muslim control were the Saracen armies which, ranging as far to the west as Gibraltar, occupied Spain, crossed the Pyrenees and seemed likely to subdue the whole of France until they were confronted and repulsed by Charles Martel at Poitiers in AD 730. The Arabs withdrew from France but brought their administrative skills and influence to bear on their Spanish province, from which they were not expelled for another three hundred years. Unfortunately, along with their religion and civilization, they brought smallpox, which remained behind after their departure and ultimately spread across France to the British Isles.

Looking for evidence of the disease's progress in England and Wales we are confronted once again by the inflexible Creighton, who asserts uncompromisingly that 'there is no independent evidence that smallpox or measles existed in England in the fourteenth and fifteenth centuries'. This opens up a large gap since the last mention of its progress on the other side of the Channel. The explanation he offers is that '[in] those times diseases were called by their external marks, so that diseases essentially most unlike but having certain spots or blemishes or pustules on the skin in common were called by a common name'. Several examples appear to confirm this view. A chart compiled by Fenner, plotting the history of smallpox 'from ancient times to 1900', includes an entry for the tenth century: 'Daughter of King Alfred of England has? smallpox' [sic]. Dixon, writing in 1962, is more specific: in AD 907 'Princess Elfrida, a daughter of [King] Alfred the Great contracted smallpox and recovered'. The source for this would appear to be James Moore who, under the same date, records that 'Princess Elfrida was sick of the smallpox and recovered'. But Moore cites no authority, and an isolated instance of the disease, preceded and followed by generations of silence, must at least give grounds for suspicion, unless of course it occurred briefly and vanished again, leaving no further record of its passage.

Other frequently quoted references to smallpox in mediaeval times have met with similar scepticism. The disease of which Gaddesden claimed to have cured a son of Edward the Third was, according to Dixon, chickenpox. An account of a 'pestilence' that allegedly caused many deaths in 1366 is shown by Creighton to have undergone transformation and amplification by various hands before Holinshed, in 1577, produced a wholly unfounded assertion that it was smallpox. On the other hand, a later historian, Goodall, asserts that 'though there is no mention of smallpox in English writings before 1518, there can be no doubt that it was prevalent in England long before that date', and gives numerous examples.

After the exploration of these and many similar byways it is a relief to reach what even the most circumspect of chroniclers is prepared to acknowledge as 'the first recorded case of smallpox in England'. The date was 22 November 1561. Master Richard Allington, believing himself to be dying, summoned various doctors of law to his bedside and addressed them: 'Maisters, seeinge that I must nedes die, which I assure you I never thought would cum to passe by this disease, considering it is but the small pockes...' Since the invalid apparently thought of his affliction as a minor one, perhaps his worst fears were not realized.

In the following year, 1562, smallpox finally established itself as a disease of the English by striking at royalty. In October, in the sixth year of her reign, Queen Elizabeth nearly died from a severe attack. The after-effects were less calamitous than many a later sufferer had to endure and according to Hopkins the long-held belief that the red wigs that the Queen wore were intended to conceal baldness must be given up. Three fellow victims met with remarkably varied fates:

> Lady Mary Sidney, who had helped to care for the ill Queen, recovered but was so disfigured that she never appeared at court again without wearing a mask. Mrs. Sibell Penn, former nurse to Edward the Sixth, died of smallpox on 6 November. Another lady of the court also recovered, apparently without severe scarring.

With smallpox finally recognized as a potentially formidable disease in its own right and with a lifetime of four hundred years ahead of it, the obvious questions arise. What sort of disease was it? How did it manifest itself? What steps were taken to control it? And above all, how did it acquire its capacity, surpassing those of almost all other maladies, to inspire dread and horror among all classes of society? Conventional accounts in fact and fiction fasten upon its possible aftermath for those lucky enough to survive an attack – disfigurement, disablement, blindness. These, though not to be brushed aside or underestimated, are the visibly striking consequences of a complex phenomenon whose strands need to be disentangled. The views of smallpox set out in what follows are, as far as possible, those which presented themselves to contemporary observers who studied and did their best to overcome it.

During the first century BC, at about the time when Julius Caesar was subduing Gaul and preparing to invade Britain, Lucretius was composing his great poem *On the Nature of Things* (or as one translation has it *On the Nature of the Universe*). From predecessors he took over the concept of

> atoms, from which nature creates all things [...] To these in my discourse I commonly give such names as the 'raw material' or 'generative bodies' or 'seeds' of things. Or I may call them 'primary particles', because they come first and everything else is composed of them.[3]

Towards the end of the work, which he did not live to complete, Lucretius embarked on an explanation of 'the nature of epidemics'.[4] He had already shown that 'there are certain atoms of many substances that are vital to us, and that on the other hand there must be countless others flying about that are pestiferous and poisonous. When these, by some chance, have accumulated and upset the balance of the atmosphere, the air grows pestiferous.' The pestilence either came from the sky like clouds and mists or sprang from the earth itself 'when it has been rotted by unseasonable drenching with unseasonable rains or pelting with sunbeams'. Different parts of the world affected by different climates produced different diseases, or the same diseases at different times.

Lucretius would have been unacquainted with smallpox but his theory of epidemic disease in general fitted in well with the observations of later writers and practitioners of medicine, who themselves must have taken their cue from the ancient Greek Hippocratic school. It was recognized that outbreaks of smallpox tended to occur at particular times of year and under certain atmospheric conditions. According to Rhazes, in tenth-century Arabia these were 'the latter end of the autumn, and the beginning of spring, and when in the summer there are great and frequent rains with continued south winds, and when the weather is warm and the winds are southerly'. Six centuries later, in Britain, Thomas Sydenham seemed to agree, although he shifted the emphasis slightly. 'This is a disease properly of the spring, [which] grows up with the heat and warmth of the year and is most severe and mortale in the sultriest part of the summer.' In a 'very epidemical year' it might 'run out in great vigor till the return of the next year'. Willan, who kept records of the atmospheric conditions in London over a long period, noted that in 1800, 'the hottest summer of any within my recollection' (he was born in 1757) 'the cases of natural small-pox were so virulent... that nearly one third of them proved fatal'.

It was natural that, in line with the doctrine of Lucretius, attempts should be made to establish a direct connection of some kind between the disease and the physical environment in which it flourished. To Rhazes the primary cause of smallpox lay in 'occult dispositions in the air', a phrase that Lucretius would surely have deplored, with its implication of some mysterious presence in the physical world which lay beyond the power of mortals to comprehend. Several centuries later Sydenham and others were accounting for smallpox with phrases such as an 'epidemical disposition' or 'peculiar constitution' of the atmosphere, which was not a great improvement on the occult, relying on the kind of circular argument familiar in other contexts. What is the cause of smallpox? An epidemic constitution of the atmosphere. What is an epidemic constitution? It is what causes smallpox.

Some authorities in due course hedged their bets. 'I do not believe,' Dimsdale wrote,

> that the state of the air, call it epidemical, or by any other name, ever generates the small-pox, unless aided by contagion, but I allow it to be true, that certain seasons and constitutions of the air are more favourable than others to spread infection, and *propagate the distemper*. [author's italics]

Woodville, while dismissing talk of 'any perceptible state of the air' as 'highly visionary and chimerical', had little to put in its place. 'The small-pox [...] seems to have originated from causes so perfectly incomprehensible as to set at defiance all rational conjecture.' Haygarth, while paying lip service to his illustrious predecessors and contemporaries, could not disguise his contempt for anything verging on the occult:

> It is allowed that this quality is produced neither by moisture nor dryness, by heat nor coldness, nor by any other sensible temperature of the air [...] While such an opinion prevails, the wildest visionary can never hope to retard the progress of this destructive malady, except by prayers or the merciful intervention of Providence. It is astonishing what implicit credit this doctrine has obtained, though positively contradicted and disproved by facts which lie open to every observer.

In spite of this forthright declaration, the doctrine of epidemic constitution was still a powerful force in the mid-nineteenth century. Gregory informed the audience at his lectures, delivered in 1842, that 'The present most approved theory of epidemic influence attributes everything to the atmosphere but [no apparatus] aids us in our researches'.

Another concept that enjoyed a long life was that of the miasm, a convenient but ill-defined entity that perhaps owed something to the 'atoms' and 'seeds' of Lucretius. Its notional function can be deduced from doubts expressed by Sutton: 'With respect to the peculiar miasm or contagious essence, whatever it may be should such a thing specifically or abstractedly exist (which as yet appears to be questionable)...' Haygarth, who might have been expected to show little respect for abstract essences, could only describe the agent that communicated smallpox, at this stage of understanding of the disease, as the 'variolous poison', or, as he expressed it elsewhere, 'Persons liable to the small-pox are infected by breathing the air, impregnated with variolous miasms...' As with epidemic constitutions, matters had progressed little further by the time of Gregory, who is found referring to 'diseases which originate from a poison or miasm – which are, as we say, "mias-matic diseases"'.

As it happened, 1842 also saw the publication of Edwin Chadwick's epoch-making *Report on the sanitary condition of the labouring population of Great Britain*, which left no doubt as to the origins of the offending miasms in the filth and squalor of the expanding manufacturing districts that were among the less admirable by-products of the Indus-trial Revolution. The consequent fixed but false assumption in some quarters that the miasmatic diseases could confidently in future be renamed 'filth diseases' helped to fuel a bitter controversy that had still not wholly died down as the nineteenth century gave way to the twentieth.

* * *

So much for the external influences that might cause patients to undergo an attack of smallpox. What of the mechanism of their own bodies that might predispose them to become victims and help them to withstand it, or not, as the case might be? For some centuries the best concept that medical men had to rely on in their attempts to deal with disease was the familiar but somewhat imprecise notion of 'the humours'. This doctrine, which exerted a strong influence in most advanced societies as late as the eighteenth century, was formulated in ancient times and taken over as the basis for the treatment of disease by the Arabian school of medical practitioners and theorists in the tenth century AD. The humours were conceived of as four bodily fluids: blood, phlegm, choler or yellow bile and melancholy, a black bile. Each of these had a different function, so that a proper balance maintained between them would ensure the physical and mental health of the individual. Conversely, an imbalance, brought about by external or internal factors, would lead to disease or emotional distress. Since both the diagnosis of a malady and the choice of remedy were largely determined in accordance with this primitive doctrine, the results were inevitably inclined to be varied and unpredictable. Sydenham, whose contribution to the treatment of smallpox came to be highly regarded for its concentration on clinical observation of the progress of the disease in individual cases rather than on uncritical acceptance of abstract theory, was, at least in this respect, uncharacteristically undogmatic:

> what this disease is in its essence I know not, nor am I able to apprehend by reason of the common and natural defects of human understanding. But never the lesse the more strict consideration inclines me to believe that it is an inflammation (though of a different species from all the others) in the blood and humours, wherein during the first three or four days, nature is intent upon the digestion of the inflamed particles, which afterwards, being amandated to the habit of the body, she further ripens and expels by way of several small abscesses.

For decades after smallpox had established itself as a serious disease there was uncertainty and confusion as to what its 'essence' might be. Two European physicians, the Belgian Van Helmont and the Dutchman Boerhaave, independently came nearest to the explanation that finally solved the riddle. Unfortunately Boerhaave muddied the waters by introducing an idea that was subsequently discredited. In the English translation of his *Aphorisms concerning the knowledge of diseases*, Boerhaave stated that smallpox,

> though epidemical, is catched from another who had it first by a contagion which at first seems to be in the air, and to be transferred into the lungs, mouth, nostrils, gullet, stomach and intestines, and consequently has yet but a small share of the poisonous quality [...] This contagious matter being mixed with the humours...

From this point the significant concept of the transmission of the disease from person to person by infection wandered off, to become lost in the mystical realm of the humours. How little impact this presumably had in Britain at the time and for some years afterwards is suggested by Frewen writing in 1749:

> The small-pox is supposed to arise from a pestilential virus or matter lodged in the blood which sooner or later being moved or acted upon by some evident cause of peculiar constitution of the air is disposed to break out on most people at one time or another, and the more early usually the better [...] the matter seems to multiply itself in the blood and augment with the patient's age.

Even as late as the 1840s, according to Gregory, 'a large proportion of mankind believe small-pox may be bred in the blood, like gout or rheumatism or independent of all direct external agency'.

For centuries following the early pronouncements of Rhazes the standard treatment for smallpox stressed the application of heat by any means that might promote it, such as the colour red. Gaddesden is chiefly famous for his claim to have cured his royal patient by wrapping him in a red cloth: 'I made everything about his bed red, and it is a good cure and I cured him in the end without marks of small-pox'. This may suggest that the sufferer's complaint was not smallpox but possibly measles or chickenpox.

The favoured heat treatment was described in detail by a Dutch physician quoted by Gregory:

> Keep the patient in a room close shut. If it be winter let the air be corrected by large fires. Take care that no cold gets to the patient's bed. Cover him well with blankets [...] never shift the patient's linen till after the fourteenth day [of the eruptive phase] for fear of striking in the pock, to the irrecoverable ruin of the patient. Far better is to let the patient bear with the stench, than to let him change his linen and thus let him be the cause of his own death [...] Sudorific [i.e. sweat-producing] expulsives are in the meantime to be given plentifully such as treacle, pearls and saffron.

This was written somewhere around 1640, shortly before Sydenham brought about one of the most significant changes in the treatment of smallpox by advocating the exact opposite, the so-called cold, or cooling regime, much to the anger of adherents to the old ways.

> How have the good ladies been offended that I have slighted their cordials and would not suffer the children who were committed to my care to die as their friends and relations had done heretofore. What stories of extravagance and folly have the talk of prejudiced people brought upon me, soe much that it has been told to persons of quality that I have taken those who had the small-pox out of their beds and put them into cold water.[5]

Sydenham's practice, at least as far as the discrete form of the disease was concerned, was broadly speaking to interfere as little as possible. 'Whoever labours under the distinct kind hardly needs the aid of the physician, but gets well of himself and by the strength of nature.' On the other hand, for the severe or confluent form of the disease he intervened actively, with a sequence of the routine measures resorted to in most cases of sickness: vomits, purges, bleeding and so on, from which even very young children were not exempt.

* * *

The generic term 'smallpox' covered what were in fact numerous strains of the virus. Gregory began his course of lectures on eruptive fevers with the announcement: 'I shall speak here of confluent, semi-confluent, carymbose, distinct and modified small-pox – of superficial, cellular and tracheal small-pox – of the benignant, malignant and petechial small-pox – of simple and complicated small-pox.' More than a century later another expert, Dixon, in what must surely rank as the most comprehensive study of the disease, identified nine varieties.

For generations of physicians who had to treat smallpox there were for practical purposes two kinds, described by Rhazes the 'good sort' and the 'bad sort'. The most significant difference between them was that the 'good', or 'distinct' (later 'discrete'), sort would probably allow you to survive, whereas the 'bad', or 'confluent', sort would almost certainly kill you. Being able to tell one from the other in good time was therefore of some importance, even though there might be nothing of significance to be done about it. William Wagstaffe, a contemporary but by no means an admirer of Lady Mary Wortley Montagu, took the most extreme view:

> There is scarcely, I believe, so great a difference between any two distempers in the world as between the best and worst of small-pox, in respect of the danger which attends them; nor perhaps is there any thing that has been more prejudicial and unfortunate to many families, than the mistakes which have arisen from their want of knowing the difference: so true is the common observation, that there is one sort which a nurse cannot kill, and another which even a physician can never cure.[6]

Presumably this meant that the most incompetent nurse could not kill her patient. What was beyond dispute was that no one, not even a skilled physician, could 'cure' him or her. As Moore explained, smallpox of any kind was a disease for which no specific remedy was known: 'When a human being is once affected with it the poison cannot be destroyed; but the disease, in spite of all medical aid, must go through its stated course.'

There are many accounts, going into more or less gruesome detail, of the progress of an attack of smallpox. Reduced to its essentials, the first stage, incubation, lasts about twelve days, during which the victim is unaware of his or her condition, and not infective until the beginning of the next or prodromal stage. This occupies a further two or three days and is marked by the onset of a fever, rising in some cases to delirium, accompanied by acute pains in various parts of the body and in some cases a rash. This leads in turn to the eruptive stage, when the fever eases a little, but the characteristic rash of spots appears in a regular sequence of time and location, beginning with the face and spreading to the rest of the body by way of the arms, the chest, the back and the legs. During the whole of this stage the patient is infectious.

Not all cases of smallpox ended fatally. Moore described the 'great variety of appearances' which the pustule might put on:

> sometimes it is very small, sometimes large and full: it generally fills with pus, but in confluent cases with lymph, and in very mild cases little or no fluid forms in the pimples. The pustules grow dry, or scab, at all periods from two days to fourteen, or more; and it is no uncommon case for the fever of the small-pox to take place without a single spot of eruption in the whole body. When to this is added, that there are a number of eruptive complaints where the pustules are extremely similar to those of the small-pox, the discrimination becomes sometimes absolutely impossible.[7]

Conversely, there was no difficulty in identifying a case of the 'bad' or confluent smallpox, of which there were numerous varieties, caused by bacterial infection of the pustules (an explanation not available, of course, to physicians during the early centuries of the incidence of the disease). The term 'confluent' implied not simply that the attack was severe, but that, in Dixon's words, 'the individual lesions [or spots] touch one another and coalesce, forming a network of lesions with small islands of unaffected skin'. Moore is here describing a case, with all its terrors, as it might be seen in a small child:

> [The] disease is usually ushered in with violent epileptic fits, which sometimes at once blast the tender infant. Should it escape this first danger, the whole body becomes covered with fiery spots, the eyelids are swollen and closed, the face grows turgid, and covered with a hard crust, rough like the bark of the elm, with cracks and fissures discharging acrid ichor. A cadaverous smell issues from the person which exhales contagion. The sufferings are inexpressible, unless delirium happily produces insensibility, and

the crisis of this deplorable state is commonly death. A few indeed struggle through, having their features disfigured with scars, or perhaps losing one or both their eyes.[8]

A modern authority, Conybeare, comments that the pustular stage of the disease, which took four or five days to complete, could result in 'the obliteration of the ordinary features' making the patient unrecognizable.

The infection of natural or 'casual' smallpox was for the most part dangerous only to those who, not yet having suffered an attack, came into close contact with the patient, and received it directly by way of the skin rash and, more particularly, the sores within the mouth and throat. However, it could be carried longer distances by clothing or bedding sent out of the house. The period of infection lasted until at least the final disappearance of the scabs, but could persist for several days in a case that had ended fatally. There was no way of telling at the beginning of an attack how serious it would prove to be: all strains of the virus were 'immunologically homogeneous',[9] but there was no explanation for the differences between mild and severe cases. The virus attacked only human beings: whatever its origin may have been in the jungles or on the grasslands of pre-history, no experiments ever succeeded in transferring it from humans to animals.

There were some characteristics of smallpox, recognized from earliest times, that appeared so nearly invariable that Gregory gave them the formal status of 'laws'. The least contentious was the 'law of non-recurrence', meaning simply that anyone who had survived one attack of smallpox was most unlikely ever to experience another; a rare second attack would in any case be so mild as barely to attract attention or cause inconvenience. This virtually certain immunity was the basis for the process of 'ingrafting', or 'inoculation', to which Lady Mary submitted her young son. The phenomenon played an essential part in the treatment of the disease since it enabled those who had survived it to tend in safety those who were passing through it. In general, to be able to point to evidence of having had smallpox was a recommendation when applying for a post such as a servant or a children's nurse. The 'law' was fundamental to any prospect of being able ultimately to 'extirpate' or eliminate the disease as a social evil. The other essential requirement was that susceptible persons, such as newborn babies or immigrants from areas where smallpox was unknown, should come face to face only with former victims – in practice an almost impossible goal before the achievement of the WHO.

Slightly more open to question was the 'law of universal susceptibility', defined as the principle, 'generally recognised' according to Gregory, that 'small-pox and measles necessarily and unavoidably occur to every man once in the course of his life'. This belief originated, or at least came to the fore, with the Arabians: 'Avicenna distinctly announces the fact and strives to account for it'. Rhazes is a little more cautious, settling for the proposition that 'hardly anyone escapes [the distemper]'. In the modern era Sydenham weighed in with the assertion that 'the small pox of all other diseases is the most common, as that which sooner or later (at least in this part of the world) attaques most men'. From that time on, for the better part of two centuries, almost every authority on the subject reiterated the assumed 'law' in their own terms. Willis, for example, combined Gregory's two laws into one: 'the escape of a man living to the ordinary period of human life from smallpox and measles is as rare as the falling into them twice'.

Susceptibility was not universal. Woodville, Gregory's predecessor at the Small Pox hospital, estimated the proportion of insusceptible children at about 1 in 60, with the figure rising to 1 in 20 among adults. This makes the 'law' as expressed somewhat misleading. From the time of the Arabians it had been accepted that the time of life when 'men' (and women) were most likely to be attacked by smallpox was earliest infancy. The truth of this observation was to some extent obscured by the circumstances in which the disease first gained ground in Britain in the sixteenth and seventeenth centuries. Reports of individual cases highlighted its steadily increasing growth among the upper classes, masking, it was alleged, whatever developments may have been taking place lower down the social ladder. Sydenham, who has been accused of being too much preoccupied with his better-off patients at the expense of the worse off, had his own sardonic explanation for the apparent preponderance of the rich victim over the poor. How did it come about

> that in the small-pox so few die amongst the common people, in comparison with the rich, which cannot be thought referable to any other cause, than that they are deprived through the narrowness of their fortunes and their rude way of living of the opportunities of hurting them selves with a more precise and tender keeping.

Another theory suggests that the disease flourished among the upper classes because they travelled more extensively than the common folk and may have brought the disease back with them from abroad.

Whatever the truth of the matter there is no lack of evidence to show that smallpox was not yet, as it subsequently became, an illness largely confined to the lower classes. Samuel Pepys, avoiding the contagion himself, recorded in his diaries the ravages wrought by the disease among the noblest families in the land. In September 1660, for example, the eleven-year-old Duke of Gloucester 'dyed of the small-pox – by the great negligence of the doctors'. On Christmas Eve 'the Princess Royal dyed at Whitehall', after only a short illness, much fault, according to Lady Sandwich, being once again laid on the doctors for not being able to decide whether the princess had smallpox, measles or spotted fever. In October 1664 the disease claimed the life of a son of Lord Derby. In 1667 it was the turn of the Duke of York, who luckily recovered, 'and blessed be God, he is not at all worse [...] but only a little weak yet'. In February 1668 'hardly ever was remembered such a season for the smallpox as these last two months have been, people being seen all up and down the streets, newly come out after the small-pox'. A month later the Duchess of Richmond was 'pretty full of the smallpox by which all do conclude she will be wholly spoiled, which is the greatest instance of the uncertainty of beauty that could be in this age'. Of another beauty whose portrait he saw, painted just before she succumbed to the disease, Pepys commented: 'it would make a man weep to see what she is like to be, by people's discourse, now.' To put this into perspective, Sydenham, referring to the same epidemic, described it as 'regular and of a mild type. It cut off comparatively few among the immense number of those who took it.'

The most prominent victim of the disease, during Pepys's last years, was Queen Mary, eulogized by Bishop Burnet, a close confidant of the royal family, by Walter Harris, Fellow of the College of Physicians and 'the personal attendant of King William and the Queen', and subsequently by Macaulay in his *History of England*. The Queen had never had smallpox, which was 'raging about London [...] in the winter of 1694'. When she was plainly sickening of something there was, according to Macaulay, the usual conflict of opinion as to the nature of the illness: '[It] was measles: it was scarlet fever: it was spotted fever: it was erysipelas.' The final diagnosis was 'small-pox of the most malignant type', although Harris, who attended her during her last days, stood firmly by his own belief that it was both smallpox and measles: 'the force of both diseases was united [...] [a union] I had more than once observed'.

Harris's first-hand account of the Queen's illness and death forms part of some 'Medical Observations on several grievous diseases' which were added to his seminal work, *A treatise of the acute diseases of infants*, written in Latin in 1697 and translated into English in 1742. The general thesis of this study conforms to the received wisdom of the period. 'As the acidity of the humours is the primary cause of all the disorders with which the tender age is wont to be tormented, the whole art of cure turns entirely in subduing the acid.' On specific disorders, '[t]he small-pox and measles of infants, which commonly are no more than mild and quiet effervescence of their blood, seldom are attended with any danger, where neither the aid of physick is called in, nor the skill of experienced nurses, as they are fancied to be, is made use of'. It might in certain cases be necessary to administer physic to relieve 'the tumult in the blood', but 'the volatile spirits in vogue, cordial waters, mithridate, Venice treacle and other hot alexipharmicks or diaphoretics are diligently to be avoided [...] such things [...] much oftener change the small-pox, which of itself was mild enough, into a dangerous sort...'

The juxtaposition in the same volume of an account of hideous death from the 'worst sort' of smallpox, along with an assurance that among infants smallpox was normally a mild and quiet affair, 'seldom attended with any danger', not only epitomizes the position at the turn of the century but also illustrates an important truth about the nature and subsequent history of the disease. Smallpox, although 'immunologically homogeneous', did not manifest itself as an unvarying feature of the epidemiological landscape. In its behaviour it had something in common with the sea. It had its tidal ebbs and flows, its periods of flat calm punctuated by violent storms, its currents, apparently constant and reliable, which could nevertheless from time to time, as a result of some external intervention, imperceptibly or startlingly change their course. Periods of low incidences gave way to epidemics of varying degrees of severity every two or sometimes four years: demographic factors such as population movements, higher birth rates or lower mortality rates disrupted the existing pattern; the introduction successively of the two prophylactics, inoculation and vaccination, especially the latter, brought about more lasting changes; fundamental variations in the virus itself may also have played their part.

Historians of the disease have charted some of the phases through which it passed. Describing its incidence in general Creighton noted that 'it first left the richer classes, then it left the village, then it left the provincial town to centre itself in the capital; at the same time it was leaving the age of infancy and childhood'. A corollary of this sequence was that, in the words of another historian, by the early nineteenth century it had become 'a disease of the poor. It did have its share of victims among the rich, but as it contracted to the great cities [it] increasingly became an infestation of the slums.' Of the eighteenth century in particular Miller concluded that 'The Age of Reason could just as truthfully be labelled the Age of Smallpox'.[10]

Smallpox was generally acknowledged to have reached its peak by about 1780, entering thereafter on a steady, though far from uninterrupted, decline: 1796, the year in which Jenner ventured on his first experiment with vaccination, also saw the highest total of deaths from smallpox for the whole century in London.

From the time towards the middle of the seventeenth century when the disease became more unsparing in its assault on the upper classes, its capacity to inspire alarm and dread among them grew in proportion while tending to decline among the lower classes. Its later reputation as a horrific and almost universal killer owed something to the unfettered imagination and descriptive powers of authors such as Macaulay, profoundly moved by the death of Queen Mary:

> That disease, over which science has since achieved a succession of glorious and beneficent victories, was then the most terrible of all the ministers of death. The havoc of the plague had been far more rapid: but plague had visited our shores only once or twice within living memory; and the small pox was always present, filling the churchyards with corpses, tormenting with constant fears all whom it had not yet stricken, leaving on those whose lives it spared the hideous traces of its power, turning the babe into a changeling at which the mother shuddered, and making the eyes and cheeks of the betrothed maiden objects of horror to the lover.

This highly wrought passage drew from Creighton the wry comment, '[i]t is not given to all of us to write like this; but it is possible that the loss of picturesqueness may be balanced by a gain of accuracy and correctness'. In fairness to Macaulay, he was dealing specifically with the era when smallpox was a new and uncontrollable hazard imposing itself impartially on rich and poor alike. Even so, Creighton had a point: as numerous passages already quoted suggest, the picture was not universally as black as Macaulay and others painted it.

It is true that throughout the eighteenth century smallpox continued to be a great destroyer of lives, but among cases of the casual or natural disease death occurred at an average rate of 1 in 6. Many who caught it in a mild form and passed through it safely avoided being disfigured, and thus turning the entire nation into a parade of grotesques. The destruction did not proceed in an unbroken sequence: during periods of perhaps a decade or so at a time, as for example between 1698 and 1710, the virus was largely quiescent. There were many parts of the kingdom in which smallpox may have been feared but was scarcely known. If there were once what might, following Gregory's example, be termed a 'law of universal horror' it steadily lost much of its relevance as time went by, for reasons having less to do with medical advances than with quirks of human nature, which emerge from the testimony of contemporary observers during the later years of the century.

Dimsdale reported a shift in the public response: 'In the earliest part of my life mankind were in general more fearful of small-pox than at present. Country people dreaded coming to town lest they should catch the distemper, and residents in town were cautious of going into the way of infection.' At about the same period Watson, writing as a medical practitioner, revealed almost casually how the profession rated the disease: 'The small-pox in its mild and distinct [i.e. discrete] state is seldom, except among persons of distinction, an object of the care of physicians in London out of hospital. They are most frequently consulted in the worst kind of disease; when it is of too considerable a magnitude to admit of much relief from the medical art.'[11]

A revealing comment on the contemporary situation was made by Haygarth in 1782 following the failure of a scheme launched in Chester with the aim of eradicating smallpox from the city:

> In Chester and I believe in most of the large towns of England the casual small-pox is almost constantly present. All the children of the middle and higher ranks of our citizens are inoculated in early infancy. The populace, very generally regarding the distemper as inevitable, neither fear nor shun it, but much more frequently by voluntary or intentional intercourse endeavour to catch the casual infection […] It is with concern we remark that in one part of the town […] the inhabitants, disregarding an inspector's exhortations, have purposely propagated the distemper, carrying the poison and even the patients, from one house to another without reserve.

As a consequence, the disease spread through fifteen families, 'infecting all in the entry [court] liable to it, and proved fatal to several'. Similar behaviour was observed in Scotland. Monro reported that

> when small pox appears favourable in one child of a family the parents generally allow commerce of their other children with the one in the disease: nay, I am assured that in some remote Highland parts of this country it has been an old practice of parents whose children have not had the small pox to watch for

an opportunity of any child of their neighbours being in good mild small pox, that they may communicate the disease to their own children by making them bedfellows to those in it, and by tying worsted threads wet with the pocky matter round their wrists.

This practice served well as long as the disease took a mild form: if not, the consequences were likely to be horrific. Another doctor, Buchan, commonly saw 'two or three children lying in the same bed with such a load of pustules that their skins stuck together'.

Various explanations have been put forward for what Haygarth called 'this strange delusion and perversity of disposition'. One of the harshest is proposed by Dixon:

Throughout the whole [eighteenth] century much of the public were content with a life of cruelty, the love of bloodsports and gambling [...] In 1748 a girl of seventeen was burnt at the stake for poisoning her mistress, and adolescents were hanged for quite minor offences. It cannot really be believed that men [and women] were particularly upset by the ravages of smallpox amongst the many risks that life held.

Contemporaries trying to control those ravages were inclined to take a more sympathetic view of the parents' problem: how to deal with children living in crowded urban conditions which made the creation of a safe environment next to impossible. In 1663, when smallpox was present in the town house of 'My Lord Hinchingbrooke', his young daughters were kindly offered sanctuary in the country home of the parents of his junior colleague, Samuel Pepys. The mass of the population had no such convenient escape route: they were literally all in it together. 'No person', Haygarth wrote,

could possibly go into an infected chamber, either on duty or by accident, but his clothes and everything around him would be rendered penitential. Nothing less than a total separation of patients in the small-pox, and all their attendants, from those who are liable to the distemper, would be sufficient security from infection. To effect this, regulations would be required that are absolutely impracticable in a free country.

In time segregation of this kind came to be accepted as both necessary and practicable, and was firmly imposed. Until that day should come perhaps the poor knew what they were doing when they tried to get their children through the disease at the age when they were least likely to come to harm from it.

A more scientific but in no sense less daunting perspective on the problem was offered by Gregory when, codifying once again the conclusions drawn by numerous observers, he propounded the 'law of vicarious mortality'. The import of this was that where the acute febrile affections – smallpox, measles, scarlet fever, erysipelas – were concerned, 'whenever one epidemic diminishes another increases', or in more sombre terms, '[e]verything teaches us that when one avenue to death is closed another opens...' Few parents, even in the moneyed and better-educated classes, were likely to come across sophisticated concepts of disease formulated in latinate phraseology: but if the experience of the lower classes taught them that, should smallpox not carry off their infants, something equally horrendous would, they could surely be forgiven for not taking the business of child-rearing too seriously.

* * *

If smallpox, long since claimed to be extinct throughout the world, survives in the folk memory, it is likely to be less because of its reputation as a killer than because of its reputation as a destroyer of good looks. Even here, as with so much else involving the disease, it is necessary to separate the truth from the hype.

In some societies, to be 'pock-marked' was to lose caste and become an object at best of compassion and at worst of disgust or even alarm, but this seems to have been a relatively late development, in limited situations. Leaving aside the horrifying spectacle of the 'worst sort' of smallpox, which almost always ended in death, the consequences of an attack were often so inconsiderable as to pass without notice, and received little attention from physicians. Rhazes offered a 'liniment which removes the marks of the smallpox', consisting of chick peas, bean meal and melon seed, and recommended 'in order to efface the pock holes and render them even with the surface of his body, let the patient endeavour to grow fat and fleshy, and use the bath frequently, and have his body well rubbed'. Gaddesden claimed that, thanks to his 'red cloth' treatment, he was able to cure his royal patient 'without marks of smallpox'. Sydenham's remedy for preserving the face from disfigurement was 'to use noe thing at all'. The oils and liniments usually prescribed 'doe retard the drying up of the ulcers, and by this delay the [poison] contained in them causes the greater excavations'. There was little danger of any mischief to the face if the patient had not been exposed to too much heat, 'and the like may be said of the eyes, putting aside the swelling of the [eyelids] which sometimes causes blindness for a little time, but is natural to the disease and needeth no other remedy saveing a little breast milk or some such slight thing to be dropped in, both to ease and moisten the part'. The sort of smallpox that occurred between Christmas and midsummer 'leaves not any impression which disfigures the face as doth very often those of the contrary season of the year'.

The general assumption at this period appears to have been that dealing with pitting could safely be left to any competent nurse. Creighton concluded a fairly lengthy study of the subject with the assertion that he had found nothing in the medical writings of the eighteenth century, nor in its fiction or memoirs, to show that pock-marks were 'more than an occasional blemish of the countenance, at a time when most sufferers had smallpox in infancy or childhood, when the chances of permanent marking would be less'. He seems to have felt some affinity with another authority who ascribed the fuss about pockmarks to women who 'set the fairness of their faces above life itself'. The jibe seems a little unkind. Standards of beauty vary from place to place and epoch to epoch. The face was especially vulnerable to disfigurement because smallpox had a strong preference for sebaceous glands, which are more common there than elsewhere, 'closely set and relatively large; [...] destruction here results in deep fibrotic pits in spite of the particular ability (of the face) in tissue repair' (Dixon). The young woman in the poem, when asked 'What is your fortune, my pretty maid?', replies 'My face is my fortune, sir', which has been suggested as a direct reference to the advantage of freedom from pockmarks.

On the other hand there is evidence that the blemishes left by the disease, as long as they were not too pronounced, were not necessarily an obstacle to matrimony. Jane Austen's brother James, a widower with a little daughter, having been turned down by his cousin Eliza, was quite happy to be accepted by the 26-year-old family friend Mary Lloyd, even though she was 'scarred with smallpox'.[12]

On the subject of scarring, contemporary references can offer unex-pected sidelights. The Reverend William Holland, vicar of Over Stowey in Somerset, notes in his diary for 11 November 1799 that 'Briffet is here to kill the sow'. The unfortunate man's face is 'sufficient to kill anything [...] absolutely furrowed with small pox' which, Holland remarks, is 'a very unusual thing in these days of innoculations'.[13]

It will not do, of course, to let the pendulum swing too far in the other direction. Towards the middle of the nineteenth century smallpox became associated predominantly with life among 'the great unwashed', and the old happy-go-lucky attitude to its visible legacy was no longer acceptable, the less so as the disease itself, apart from occasional outstanding episodes, began to pass from the scene. Prejudice in matters of this kind can be distressingly long-lived. Dixon reports a case as late as 1953 in which a patient recovering from a mild attack, with scarcely visible marks, was turned away from a convalescent home in Lancashire because the Medical Officer of Health, while admitting that he considered the man not contagious, was 'very much concerned as to the effect on the minds of people who are at present in residence in the home'.[14]

CHAPTER 3

THE ENGRAFTED DISTEMPER

By contrast with their outward passage the Wortley Montagus began their homeward journey by sea, admiring the landscapes and antiquities of the Mediterranean shores and islands along the way. But progress in the days of sail, in a naval vessel which had seen better times, was slow, and on reaching Genoa in August 1718 the parents decided to complete their journey overland, leaving their children, then aged respectively six and one, aboard ship with their nurse to face the winter storms of the Bay of Biscay and the English Channel. It was five months before the family was reunited on English soil.

Before leaving Constantinople, Lady Mary had written to Sarah Chiswell announcing her intention of bringing inoculation – 'this useful invention' – into fashion in England. A suitable opportunity to begin the campaign might have been the severe epidemic of smallpox that broke out in 1719, shortly after the family's return, but more pressing needs – such as finding somewhere to live – intervened. A further epidemic, only slightly less severe, occurred in 1721 and this time there was no hesitation. In April Maitland, now living in the country near London, was sent for and, in spite of a certain natural reluctance to perform on his home ground under the professional scrutiny of his peers, was prevailed upon to inoculate Edward's young sister Anne, who became the first patient to undergo the operation in England. Important personages, including some of Lady Mary's *bêtes noires* among the doctors, were privately invited (by one account 'appointed') to observe how little she had been incommoded by it – rather less so indeed than her mother, who was soon complaining of being so much harassed by people wanting to learn more about inoculation that she wanted to 'run into the country to hide myself'. One of the medical witnesses, Dr James Keith, two of whose sons had died of smallpox, was so much impressed by what he saw that he immediately asked Maitland to perform the operation on his only surviving child who had not had smallpox.

It was from one point of view Lady Mary's misfortune to have launched into her crusade – if that is not too strong a word – at a time of sharp division both within the medical profession over other matters, and in court circles at the highest level. It was a characteristic of all the Hanoverian monarchs that each should be on bad terms with his putative successor. George the First couldn't bear the sight of his son Frederick, Prince of Wales, or his daughter-in-law, Princess Caroline of Anspach, both of whom reciprocated the King's sentiments; the allegiances of the court and the upper classes in general were similarly divided. Lady Mary's position seems to have been ambiguous. She got on quite well with the King because he spoke no English and was past the age of learning it, whereas she had learned sufficient German to be able to converse with him. At the same time she was reported to share many of the intellectual interests of Frederick and Caroline, among them the subject of inoculation. A question much debated is how far Lady Mary was implicated in the decision of Princess Caroline to have two of her daughters inoculated, a step which, if successful, would raise the operation from being a matter of purely private concern to an issue of national significance. Did Lady Mary, as was and still is held in some quarters, encourage her 'friend' Princess Caroline to press ahead with her project, or did the Princess achieve her objective mostly with help from a different quarter altogether?

However cordial their relationship at a public level, Lady Mary privately had a poor opinion of the royal family. In an account of the court of George the First, probably written before she left for Constantinople but not published until some time after her death, she dismissed the whole lot of them in her famously acerbic style. The King was 'an honest blockhead [...] more properly dull than lazy', and would have stayed in Hanover if they had let him. 'Our customs and laws were all mysteries to him, which he neither tried to understand, nor was capable of understanding if he had endeavoured it.' Prince Frederick had a fiery temper, 'which being unhappily under the direction of a small understanding was every day throwing him under some indiscretion [...] he looked on all men and women he saw as creatures he might kiss or kick for his diversion...' His wife, the Princess, had 'that genius which qualified her for the government of a fool and made her despicable in the eyes of all men of sense: I mean a low cunning which gave her an inclination to cheat all the people she conversed with...' There was much more of this in the same vein. As a wit Lady Mary could hold her own with the likes of Swift, Pope and Congreve, but it is difficult to believe that she could have sustained a warm friendship with a woman whom she so comprehensively despised, and this must cast some doubt on the likelihood of her having played a leading part in the Princess's plans; which is not to say that she may not have lent any assistance within her power.

The inoculation of the young princesses was not achieved until almost a year after that of Lady Mary's daughter, during which time controversy over the danger and value of the operation gathered pace, partly because of the possible involvement of the royal family. A suggestion was put forward that the King might be asked to agree that a few condemned criminals should receive a royal pardon in return for taking part in a formal trial of inoculation under the strictest supervision. He gave his consent and, after another understandable show of reluctance, Maitland was persuaded by the royal physician, Sir Hans Sloane, to carry out the experiment, which took place in Newgate Gaol in August 1721 against a background of intense public interest. Various accounts were published, some less inaccurate than others, the most circumstantial being a pamphlet by Maitland himself, which appeared the following February.[1]

On 9 August at nine o'clock in the morning six volunteers – Mary North, aged 36; Anne Tompion, 25; Elizabeth Harrison, 19; John Cawthery, 25; John Alcock, 20; and Richard Evans, 19 – having undergone a regime of purging and other preparations during the preceding days, were handed over to Maitland. Under the watchful eyes of two dozen or so distinguished physicians, including Sloane, Maitland made incisions in both arms and the right leg of each of the six. After two days, with little to show for this, and 'suspecting the matter ingrafted to have been defective and languid', he sent out for a fresh supply, which was only sufficient for five of the party; the sixth volunteer, Richard Evans, turned out to have had smallpox in prison in the previous year.

By the middle of the following week the five were showing signs of smallpox, not particularly seriously but somewhat earlier than would have been expected in a case of the casual disease. By the end of a fortnight they were clearly tending to become uncooperative. On Saturday night 'Alcock unaccountably pricks and opens all the pustules he could come at with a pin: which occasions them to fall and crust sooner'; on Monday 'Mary North before she was quite free [of pustules] unaccountably wash'd in cold water, and thence caught a violent colic which lasted two days'. On 6 September, when the trial had been in progress for nearly a month, 'they were all dismissed to their several counties and habitations'. A short time later, one of the observers, Dr Richard Mead, obtained permission to try on a seventh prisoner, a young woman of about 18, the practice attributed to the Chinese of powdering some dried crusts of pustules and thrusting them up the nose; she suffered a more painful reaction than any of the others.

This more or less successful experiment should have answered Caroline's doubts as to the dangers of inoculation although not, of course, its possible long-term benefits, but in spite of the examples provided by the Wortley Montagu children she needed further reassurance. She 'procured' half a dozen charity children and had them inoculated. The results were satisfactory except in the case of one small volunteer 'who had had the smallpox before, tho' pretended not, for the sake of the reward'.

A different version of this sequence of events relies on a document that is unfortunately less reliable than it might have been. In February 1756 the Royal Society heard a reading of 'an account of inoculation' written by Sir Hans Sloane, 'given to Mr Ranby to be published, Anno 1736', and subsequently published in the *Philosophical Transactions*. Why it was written fifteen years after the events it describes, why it had to wait a further twenty years to be published, and where it had been in the meantime are questions to which there appear to be no completely satisfactory answers.

Lady Mary's most recent biographer accepts the paper as having been written 'at the time' (i.e. in 1721). 'The underlying facts [...] are that one of Princess Caroline's daughters had nearly died of smallpox, and that the mother to secure her other children and for the common good begged the lives of six condemned criminals for the experiment.'[2] Against this version, it was later established that the young princess's ailment had been not smallpox but scarlet fever: if it had been smallpox, the argument goes, her two younger sisters would almost infallibly have caught it from her and their own subsequent inoculation would have been pointless. Further, there appears to be a discrepancy in Sloane's own recollection, according to which it was not until *after* the experiments on the convicts and the children had taken place that the Princess of Wales sent for him 'to ask my opinion of the inoculation of the princesses', and after resolving that it should be undertaken, 'ordered me to go to the late [*sic*] King George the First who had commanded me to wait upon him upon that occasion'.

On the basis of this assertion Miller, who in other respects supports 1736 as the date of Sloane's document, concludes that 'Lady Mary's rôle in influencing the royal family in England has been exaggerated', and that 'if any one single individual ought to be singled out as *the* most influential agent in promoting the medical innovation called inoculation in England Sloane should be seriously considered [...] One sees [his] hand in every move that was made...' She considers that he exercised great tact when consulted by the Princess, although to less committed observers it may seem that what he exercised was not so much tact as the smooth equivocation of the skilled courtier:

> I told her royal highness that [inoculation] seemed to be a method to secure people from the great dangers attending the distemper in the natural way [...] but that not being certain of the consequences that might happen I would not persuade nor advise the making trials upon patients [i.e. the princesses] of such importance to the public.

Would he then *dissuade* her? 'To which I made answer that I would not, in a matter likely to be of such advantage'.[3] Similarly, when he faced the King, 'I told his majesty my opinion: that it was impossible to be certain, but that raising such a commotion in the blood, there might happen dangerous accidents not foreseen'. The King replied to the effect that people had died in similar circumstances after cases of treatment, however much care was taken. 'I told his majesty I thought this to be the same case, and the matter was concluded upon...' One is reminded of the conjurer's skill in 'forcing' a card upon an innocent volunteer.

Whoever deserves credit for pushing the matter along, the two princesses were successfully inoculated on 17 April 1722, not by Maitland but, as befitted their station, by Amyand, surgeon to the King. By this date battle had been seriously joined between supporters and opponents of the operation, and Lady Mary was bound to be in the thick of it. A highly coloured view of the scene was set down some years later by her youngest granddaughter. Lady Louisa Stewart was only five years old when her grandmother died in 1761 and was hardly likely, writing in 1837, to have recalled remarks made to her in person more than seventy years earlier about events that had occurred forty years earlier still. A possible source might be Lady Mary's diary, which came into the hands of her daughter Lady Bute (Maitland's second inoculee), who destroyed it, but not before granting a sight of it to her own daughter, Lady Louisa. Whatever their provenance the views expressed reveal the would-be benefactor of her fellow countrymen in a mood of bitter disillusionment.

According to this account, Lady Mary protested that in the four or five years immediately following her return from Constantinople

> she seldom passed a day without repenting her patriotic undertaking, and she vowed that she would never have attempted it if she had foreseen the vexation and persecution and even the

obloquy it brought upon her. The clamour raised against the practice, and of course against her, were beyond belief. The faculty [i.e.
the medical profession] all rose in arms to a man, foretelling
failure and the most disastrous consequences; the clergy descanted
from their pulpits on the impiety of others seeking to take events
out of the hands of Providence; the common people were taught
to hoot at her as an unnatural mother, who had risked the lives of
her children.[4]

The hostility of the doctors, their unwillingness to see her daughter's
inoculation succeed, was so great, Lady Mary maintained, that 'she
never cared to leave the child alone with them one second lest it should
in some way suffer from their interference'. This suggests something
approaching paranoia, and need not be taken too seriously. Lady
Mary's lifelong contempt for 'the faculty' is well documented and may
well have communicated itself to her descendants.

* * *

Looking back from the end of the century on the events surrounding
the introduction of inoculation, Woodville summarized the activities of
the opposing parties and laid on both sides blame for its failure to
produce 'the distinct or favourable kind of small-pox'. The inoculators
were at first unwilling to acknowledge the shortcomings of inoculation
'and by attempting to attribute the deaths of persons inoculated to
other accidental causes exposed themselves to just censure'. At the
same time the writers against inoculation pursued a course of conduct
even more reprehensible:

> Instead of waiting to ascertain such facts as might have enabled
> them to form just conclusions on the advantages and disadvan-
> tages of this new art they immediately proceeded to employ
> falsehood and invective, reproaching the inoculators with the
> epithets of poisoners and murderers.

The fiercest hostilities were confined to little more than the year
1722. Specific dates are not always easy to come by but there is no
doubt about the most vociferous objector, the Revd Edmund Massey,
who, on Sunday 8 July, preached in St Andrews, Holborn, *A sermon
against the dangerous and sinful practice of inoculation*. Choosing his text
from the book of Job 2.7 – 'So went Satan forth from the presence of
the Lord and smote Job with sore boils from the sole of his foot unto his

crown' – Massey suggested that Job may have been the victim of smallpox, the inference being, in Woodville's words, that 'the devil was the first inoculator and poor Job his first patient'. Massey's own gloss on the text was that since Job's sufferings, although inflicted on him by Satan, were designed by God as a test of his faith, all disease was designed by God for the same purpose, as 'a trial of our faith or the punishment of our sins'. Inoculation was therefore 'a diabolical operation which usurps an authority founded neither in the laws of nature or religion, [and] tends in this case to anticipate and banish Providence out of this world and promotes the encrease [*sic*] of vice and immorality'. Inoculators were 'diabolical sorcerers, hellish venefici, enemies of mankind'; the 'confessed miscarriages' of their new method were 'more than have happened in the ordinary way', an assertion not borne out by any figures that were currently available.

In spite of Lady Mary's allegations, dutifully reproduced by her granddaughter, religious objections to inoculation seem to have faded away fairly quickly: no clerical outburst approached the venom of Massey's. The opposition of the medical profession was more sustained and less easy to deal with. One of the earliest examples was *Reasons against the Practice of Inoculating the Small-Pox* by the surgeon Ledgard Sparham, whose arguments were founded reasonably enough on medical principles generally accepted in his day. 'The instilling of poison into a wound has always been accounted the most destructive of any: for though the blood thus fermented may betray itself in the shape of the small-pox, yet it has always a resort to a poisonous fountain, from which it may every moment receive new supplies.' Therefore the 'poison' introduced by inoculation will always produce 'effects answerable to its nature', and however often the process is repeated,

> the pustules thrown out by this new method [...] will cause the same symptoms either to those who have suffered by the natural or artificial pox. Nor can reason justify the contrary, for the condition of this matter, thus infused, will always be the same [and] unless we could suppose some singular virtue to remain in the blood as a proper antagonist it would be absurd to think them secure from a second infection....

Unfortunately this cool and, for its time, logical statement of a problem that continued to baffle medical science for the next two hundred years had to be rounded off with a volley of invective against the inoculators, by whose 'mercenary artifice' healthy people were 'persuaded to change their sound condition for a diseased one: their expectation of one day falling ill for a certain sickness now, under pretence of future security...' The life of everyone thus inoculated 'is as eminently in danger as is those who suffer from [smallpox] in the accidental way [...] Our condition is desperate and these gentlemen, these new operators, are kindly furnishing us with the materials for our despatch.'

This melancholy conclusion was shown to be false within a few years, but in the meantime a more doughty opponent of inoculation came forward, by general consent the most formidable of them all. William Wagstaffe, Fellow of the Royal Society and the College of Physicians, and a physician of St Bartholomew's Hospital, had been one of the experts invited to observe both Anne Wortley Montagu after her inoculation and the conduct of the Newgate experiment, on which he set down his own impressions. He now entered the fray with a blast on the trumpet that only the deaf or the congenitally indifferent could ignore, one that still reverberates in some quarters today. His protest took the form of *A letter to Dr Freind* [sic] *shewing the danger and uncertainty of inoculating the small pox*:

> Sir,
>   Tho' the fashion of inoculating the small pox has so far prevail'd as to be admitted to the greatest families, yet I entirely concur with you in the opinion that, till we have fuller evidence of the success of it, both with regard to the security of the operation, and the certainty of preventing the like distemper from any other cause, physicians at least, who of all men ought to be guided chiefly by experience, shou'd not be over hasty in encouraging the practice, which does not seem as yet sufficiently supported either by reason or by fact [...] Other people may be satisfied with being told that the operation is successful, but physicians, I shou'd think, cannot with prudence give into any thing which is the peculiar subject of their profession merely because it has been cry'd up by those who are no physicians and have not the least knowledge of distempers.

This was forthright and fair comment from one professional to another: it was the succeeding paragraph which put the author into the select class of chauvinists whose sins shall not be forgiven them. Casting a supercilious glance at 'the country from whence we deriv'd this experiment' Wagstaffe remarked that '[p]osterity perhaps will scarcely be brought to believe that a method practiced [sic] only by a few illiterate women, amongst an illiterate and unthinking people, shou'd on a sudden, and upon a slender experience, so far obtain in one of the most learned and polite nations of the world, as to be received into the royal palace'.

This assessment, written perhaps with his tongue some way into his cheek, has earned for Wagstaffe from a modern commentator the verdict that he was 'in today's terms racist, anti-feminist and orientalist'. But today's terms are not necessarily the best guides to the past's thinking and may be positively misleading. Stripping away a few layers of hindsight and making allowance for the indignation of a man with a possibly over-developed gift for rhetoric may reveal, to his way of thinking, genuine cause for complaint.

Wagstaffe was prejudiced but he made some pertinent criticisms. A short account of Maitland, contributed to the *Aberdeen University Review* in 1929, remarked apropos of the inoculation of young Edward Wortley Montagu that '[t]he experience of the little fellow would horrify a modern vaccinator'. Would Wagstaffe not have equal reason to be horrified by Maitland's account? With all his own shortcomings, which he shared with his contemporaries, he was a professional and could hardly help looking askance at old Greek women, emerging from one of the most remote backwaters of Europe with what sounded like some sort of folk remedy imparted, as one of them claimed, by 'the Holy Virgin', and involving walnut shells full of 'the best sort of smallpox', the ripping open of veins with blunt and rusty needles and the insertion of the noxious matter into apparently healthy bodies. There were sufficient differences between the 'natural' or 'casual' smallpox and the 'ingrafted distemper', as Wagstaffe had ascertained in Newgate, to raise some doubts at that time as to whether there was any genuine affinity between them, and therefore any solid ground for accepting that the inoculated disease could provide a lasting defence against the natural disease. On the contrary, as Maitland and his fellow inoculators soon learned to their consternation, the inoculated disease could give rise to the most severe form of the natural disease in anyone who had not yet had it. This disadvantage remained a constant source of bewilderment. Forty or more years later Dimsdale, the most successful and widely respected inoculator of his day, asked in great perplexity, 'How comes it that matter taken from inoculated patients conveys the distemper with equal certainty as if it were taken from the natural small-pox?' In modern times, when the phenomenon was no longer of any consequence, it remained the subject of speculation and hypothesis.

In early years even the basic techniques for carrying out inoculation were left more or less to the operator's fancy, perhaps because of an inadequate supply of walnut shells. A favourite method, mentioned for the first time in a lecture given in 1721 by Harris to the College of Physicians, described 'the manner of inoculation by a thread imbued with the variolous pus and rubbed on a puncture'. Pylarini, widely held to be the most reliable authority on the Byzantine operation, mentioned that it was sometimes performed on the forehead, at the base of the hair, on one side of the cheek or on the chin.

The situation with regard to inoculation in 1722, as Wagstaffe summarized it, was that '[s]ome have had the distemper not at all, others to some degree, others the worst sort and some have died of it'. This was undoubtedly a prejudiced view, unsupported by concrete evidence, but Woodville, looking back more objectively from the end of the century, commented unfavourably on Maitland's 'flattering promise' that inoculation, as practised at Constantinople, was 'a process which almost universally produced a small-pox in the mildest form, insomuch that not one person in many thousands died under it'.

The significant words were 'in Constantinople', because the truth was that, apart from Maitland himself, none of the practitioners who so eagerly undertook the novel operation had seen it performed in what might pass for the authentic manner, and were introducing their own variations. One enthusiastic convert, Dr Nettleton of Halifax, who soon had upwards of forty 'insitions' to his credit, described his procedure in a letter which found its way into the *Philosophical Transactions*:

> The method, which I always took in the operation, was to make two incisions, one in the arm and another in the opposite leg. It is not material as to raising the distemper whether the incisions be large or small; but I commonly found that, when they were pretty large the quantity of matter discharged afterwards at those places was greater, and that the more plentiful that discharge, the more easy the rest of the symptoms generally are...

The incisions, as recommended by another authority, would usually be made 'with a small lancet in the brawny part of the arm or leg, cutting just into or at most through the cutis or true skin for the length of a quarter of an inch, half an inch or at most an inch'. Into this incision matter taken from one of the donor's pustules by means of a couple of 'pledgets' of lint or cotton would be transferred and the wound covered with a plaster for a day or so.

Accounts of this kind, with their suggestion of 'the more the easier', prompted the publication of an anonymous pamphlet attributed to a 'Turkey Merchant', castigating the English physicians and surgeons for their potentially damaging methods and restating the proper procedure.[5]

This did not differ greatly from Maitland's description, but the author was at pains to emphasize, with much sarcastic comment directed at the English profession, the essential simplicity of the Greek method:

> The old nurse who is the general surgeon upon the occasion at Constantinople takes [the matter] in a nutshell which holds enough to infect 50 people, contrary to the infamous practice here, which is to fill the blood with such a quantity of that matter as often endangers the life and never fails of making the distemper more violent than it need be.

The point was that the old Greek women knew when to let well alone: 'leaving nature to herself [they] never fail of the good success which generally follows the rational way of acting', in contrast to English physicians,

> [who] must give me leave to tell them [...] that their long prepa-rations [purging, bleeding, etc.] only destroy the strength of the body necessary to throw off the infection. The miserable gashes that they give people in their arms may endanger the loss of them, and the vast quantity they throw in of that infectious matter may possibly give them the worst kind of small pox, and the cordials they pour down their throats may encrease the fever to such a degree as may put an end to their lives.

The authorship of the article remained a mystery for two hundred years until the 'Turkey Merchant' was revealed by Halsband to be Lady Mary Wortley Montagu. Its general tone was all of a piece with her known antipathy to the medical profession, but it is ironic that on this occasion she was, by implication, underlining some of Wagstaffe's crit-icisms which, by implication, had been directed at her.

CHAPTER 4

THE LANGUAGE OF FIGURES

By the end of 1722 the mutual recriminations of the opposing parties had largely died away, chiefly for want of accurate information on which to base their contradictory claims. There was clearly a need for research, conducted at a responsible level, to establish a few reliable facts at least with regard to the success or otherwise of the operation. In December 1723, and in a slightly amended form in 1724, the *Philosophical Transactions* carried an advertisement:

> The practice of inoculating the small pox being now extended into many parts of the Kingdom, and it being highly requisite that the public should be faithfully inform'd of the success of that method, whether good or bad: it is desir'd that all physicians, surgeons, apothecaries, and others therein concern'd will be pleas'd to transmit to Dr Jurin, Secretary to the Royal Society, a particular account specifying the name and age of every person by them inoculated, the place where it was done, the manner of the operation, whether it took effect or no, what sort of distemper it produced, on what day from inoculation the eruption appear'd, and lastly, whether the patient died or recover'd. They are desir'd to comprehend in their accounts all persons inoculated by them from the beginning of the practice among us to the end of the present year, and to send them some time in January or February next...

The results were to be made available to the public and to any gentleman, but the names of the persons inoculated would not be printed without their consent. The original accounts were to be preserved so that 'in case any of those who have been inoculated shall afterwards have the small pox in the natural way it may be known whether such person had before received the small pox by inoculation or not'.

Jurin had already been engaged in correspondence with Nettleton on fundamental questions such as 'whether the distemper raised by inoculation is really the small pox and [whether] it is much more mild than the natural sort'. He had himself supplied a friend from the College of Physicians with details of 182 persons inoculated up to the date of the advertisement and with the results of a comparison between the danger of natural smallpox and of that given by inoculation (*A Letter to the Learned Dr Caleb Colesworth FRS…*). Consulting the bills of mortality from 1667 onwards he found that 'upwards of seven per cent, or somewhere more than a fourteenth part of mankind die of the small pox', and since it was notorious that great numbers of young children died of other diseases without ever having smallpox it was plain that 'fewer than thirteen must recover from this distemper for one that died of it'. Various other factors, explored in the letter at some length, complicated the computation, but the result, if the situation continued in the future as in the past, was

> That of all the children there will, some time or other, die of the small pox one in fourteen;
>
> That of the persons of all ages taken ill of the natural small pox there will die of that distemper one in five or six, or two in eleven;
>
> That of persons inoculated with the same caution in the choice of subjects as has been used by the several operators one with another […] (if we allow that in two cases the persons died of the inoculated small pox) there will die one in ninety one. But if those two persons died of other diseases, then we shall have reason to think that none at all will die of inoculation, provided that proper caution be used.

Later, in the first of several annual accounts of 'the success of inoculating the small pox' (this one 'humbly dedicated to her Royal Highness the Princess of Wales'), Jurin reduced the issues to two:

1. Whether the distemper given by inoculation be an efficient security to the patient against his having the small pox afterwards in the natural way?

2. Whether the hazard of inoculation be considerably less than that of the natural small pox?[1]

The answer to the first question was that 'there is no instance, as far as I have been able to learn, of any person […] that has received the small pox by inoculation that has afterwards had it in the natural way…'; but of course 'we are not certain that the small pox does never, tho' perhaps exceedingly rarely, happen twice naturally to the same person'; and 'inoculation, like all applications in physic or surgery, will not always produce the intended effect'.

Jurin received a great many responses to his advertisements and many commentators are disposed to credit him, along with Lady Mary (or Hans Sloane, as the case may be), with having assured the widespread acceptance of inoculation. Others have pointed to errors in his statistical methods, and Creighton was inclined to dismiss even his main conclusion as a statement of the obvious, derived mostly from the labours of Nettleton.

In spite of, or perhaps because of, the controversy that attended its arrival in Britain inoculation made fairly slow progress for several years, and it was possible to keep track of most of the principal practitioners and their work rate. Up to the end of 1722 there were approximately 186 operations undertaken by thirteen known inoculators, among whom the most assiduous were Nettleton with a tally of 61 and Maitland with 57, only one other reaching double figures. In 1723 the total rose to 292, but in 1724 it dropped to 40, only Amyand getting into double figures with 11. In 1725 and 1726 the league leaders continued to be Amyand, Maitland and Nettleton, with a combined score of 256, among which there were, in Creighton's words, 'four deaths of somewhat conspicuous persons'. 1728 produced the lowest number of the decade, a mere 37. The total for eight years was 897, with 17 acknowledged deaths, after which, unless some operations somehow escaped notice, the practice seems to have fallen into desuetude for at least a further decade, and the controversy with it. Woodville noted that from 1728 to 1738 'the subject of inoculation seems to have been almost disregarded...'; the number of inoculations was 'so inconsiderable that it excited no jealousy in the anti-inoculators'.

Various reasons were suggested for the decline. Jurin, in one of his 'accounts', may have come close. 'People do not easily come into a practice in which they apprehend any hazard unless they are frightened into it by a greater hazard.' The Revd John Hough, writing towards the end of the 1730s, came even closer. Most inoculations were performed on young children. The reason why 'the method loses ground' was, in Hough's view, that 'parents are tender and fearful, not without hope that their children may escape the [natural] disease, or have it favourably: whereas [...] in the way of art [i.e. inoculation] should it prove fatal they could never forgive themselves'. Similar anxieties over immunization are not unknown among parents in modern times.

* * *

The compilation of reasonably accurate statistics showing the number of inoculations carried out per annum was a fairly simple task in the early days, given the readiness of the profession to respond to Jurin's advertisements. A much more taxing problem was the collection of reliable information on topics of wider significance: how much natural smallpox was there about at any one time, and how many people of all ages were dying of it? Jurin arrived at some plausible answers but they depended on the credibility of a system of fact-finding that was generally felt to leave a lot to be desired.

It had its origins in the reign of Queen Elizabeth. In 1592 it was decreed that the minister of every London parish should make a weekly return of the burials, baptisms and marriages recorded in his parish register. In 1604 the Company of Parish Clerks began compiling lists of deaths, classifying them according to causes, and from 1629 their tables were printed and published annually as the London bills of mortality. The only compilation of their kind throughout the country, the bills appeared without interruption and only occasional refinements until 1839, thirty-eight years after the institution of the first national census. William Farr, the compiler of abstracts at the Register Office (set up by the Registration Act of 1836), provided a brief summary of the system in a report to the Registrar General in 1864, as part of a review of the office of coroner.

The source of the information set out in the bills was a body of persons known as 'searchers' who were appointed 'to view the bodies of all those that died before they were suffered to be buried and to certify of what probable disease each individual died'. For a more detailed explanation of the 'mechanism' by which the system worked, Farr drew on an account by an earlier statistician, John Graunt, who had published some 'Observations' between 1662 and 1674:

> When anyone dies, then, either by tolling or ringing of a bell, or by bespeaking of a grave to a sexton, the same is known to the searchers, corresponding with the said sexton. The searchers hereupon (who are ancient matrons sworn to their office) repair to the place where the dead corps lies, and by view of the same, or by other enquiries they examine by what disease or casualty the corps died. Hereupon they make their report to the parish clerk, and he, every Tuesday night, carries in an accompt of all the burials and christenings happening that week to the Clerk of the Hall.

By Thursday the account was made up, published 'and dispersed to the several families who will pay four shillings per annum for it'.

The bills of mortality, which almost from the beginning had paid more attention to smallpox and plague than to other diseases, inevitably played a significant rôle in the developing controversy over the pros and cons of inoculation, incurring a good deal of criticism. As early as 1720 Richard Mead, probably the most successful and affluent physician of the day, protested that '[i]nstead of ignorant old women who are generally appointed as searchers [...] the office should be committed to understanding and diligent men...' Isaac Massey, an apothecary and uncle to the Revd Edmund, complained in a letter to Jurin that

> These bills are founded on the ignorance or skill of the old women [...] [whose] reports, (very often what they are bid to say) must necessarily be very erroneous. Many distempers which prove mortal are mistaken for the small-pox [...] yet it is generally put down by the searchers as small-pox, especially if they are told the deceased never had them.

The sexist campaign was kept going: a century later a certain Dr Burrows described diseases as specified in the bills as 'a disgrace to the medical science and civilization in which as a nation we are acknowledged to be pre-eminent'. The two old women appointed by the churchwardens, as soon as they heard 'the knell for the dead' repaired to the sexton of the parish to learn the residence of the deceased.

> They demand admittance to the house [...] and *judge* of what the person died [...] The regular charge for the performance of this office is 4d. to each searcher; but if an extra gratuity be tendered they seldom pass the threshold or hall of the house and are content with whatever account is given; or should they actually view the corpse, it is easy to imagine what credit is due to the judgment they pronounce.[2]

It was generally accepted that since the great majority of deaths occurred among children below the age of ten, in the crowded slums where they had spent their short lives, their departure could easily escape the notice of the none-too-vigilant searchers.

The 'ancient matrons' had their defenders. Graunt, while admitting that the reports might occasionally need amending, argued that many of the verdicts were a matter of common sense – you could hardly mistake a death from 'flux', or confluent smallpox, and in any case the searchers were 'able to report the opinion of the physician who was with the patient'. Farr quotes this assertion with approval, on the ground that 'there could be no doubt of the value of even the imperfect report of facts in the early bills directly concerning the life and death of Englishmen'.

The performance of the searchers might have been acceptable in the undemanding days of Charles the Second but even Farr must have recognized their unacceptable inadequacy in the reigns of William the Fourth and Victoria. It was not merely that the clerks in some parishes made returns irregularly and sometimes not at all. Even in the best-run parishes many deaths went unrecorded because the deceased, not being members of the established church, were not the concern of the minister or his clerks. Dissenters, papists and Jews had their own burial grounds; many even of the wealthy class, when they died, were removed from London for burial in the country beyond the metropolis and so escaped mention in the bills.

One aspect of the system was perhaps the source of greater statistical distortion than all the others put together. The population of London was expanding at a great rate throughout the eighteenth century, especially during the latter half, yet the geographical area on which the statistics were based remained what it had always been, the London metropolitan district, which excluded some of the most rapidly growing and increasingly overcrowded parishes, such as Marylebone or Pancras, where the Smallpox and Foundling hospitals were situated. The extent of the discrepancy was for many years a matter of guesswork, but was clearly revealed in 1801 when the results of the first national census were analysed. Giving evidence to a parliamentary inquiry Sir Gilbert Blane quoted some figures. 'The total population of the metropolis according to these returns is 864,845, of whom 117,802 are in parishes not comprehended in the bills of mortality [...] One parish alone is found to contain 63,000 inhabitants not included in the bills.'[3]

Misrepresentation of the mortality among Londoners was serious enough, but even worse were the attempts of amateur statisticians to extrapolate the figures to take in the whole country. Giving evidence to the same inquiry as Blane, a prominent physician produced a bizarre result that others copied. Admitting what everyone knew, that the London bills were defective, Lettsom took the population of the metropolis to be nearly a million, of whom it was estimated, again on the basis of the bills, that 3,000 persons died every year from smallpox; then, 'allowing Great Britain and Ireland to contain 12,000,000 of people no less than 36,000 of our fellow subjects are annually sacrificed by the small-pox'.[4] A simple matter of arithmetic, as long as it was assumed that smallpox was spread evenly throughout the country. But the truth was that although more or less endemic in the seething slums of London and possibly a few other major cities, smallpox often passed by the less densely populated areas of the country for long periods, even at the height of its prevalence in the latter part of the eighteenth century. Edwardes mentions a village in Yorkshire in which, from 1747 to 1756, out of 107 deaths only one was ascribed to smallpox; again, between 1757 and 1766 there were 212 baptisms, 156 deaths, but only 13 by smallpox. Hughes quotes a letter written in 1781 by a parent living in Gateshead: 'You will hardly credit that in this populous country Ingham has in vain searched for a patient with the small pox from whom he might procure matter to inoculate his own, our little boy and theirs'. At the other end of the country a parson in a remote parish in the Isle of Purbeck reported in 1803 that 'the visitation of small pox is a stranger, having occurred only twice in forty years, once by infection, and once by inoculation'.

Haygarth quoted from a letter addressed to him in 1782 by a cleric living in Kent:

> I have been twenty years curate of two country parishes not six miles distant from [Maidstone] [...] Boughton, about a year ago, contained [...] four hundred and ninety-seven inhabitants [...] and Hunton four hundred and thirty-two. During [...] twelve years in the former and eight in the latter, the number of deaths by the small-pox, in both, had not exceeded five [...] there have not been above five deaths in my native parish, although it now contains six hundred and twenty-four people [...] [the] annual fatality has not exceeded one in twenty thousand...

Even in the larger cities of the kingdom deaths from smallpox occurred on nothing like the scale postulated by Lettsom, Blane and others. In 1773 Haygarth recorded that 'the average of deaths by the small-pox in Liverpool is 220, in Manchester 98, in Chester 63', a total of 381.

In spite of evidence of this kind, which a little diligence would have uncovered from many quarters, what one might call the Lettsom hypothesis continued to hold the field, and even to proliferate like some noxious weed. The report of the inquiry whose members had heard Lettsom's estimate of 36,000 deaths per annum confidently asserted, '*It is proved* [report's italics] that in these United Kingdoms [...] 45,000 persons die annually of the small-pox...' The bills of mortality themselves were not proof against an arbitrary inflation rate imposed on them from outside. James Moore, who later became the Director of the National Vaccine Establishment, put the number of deaths within the bills in 1806 at 'upwards of two thousand'. The annual reports of the NVE from time to time improved upon these figures; in 1826: 'when we reflect that before the introduction of vaccination the average number of deaths from smallpox in London was annually about 4,000'; in 1836: '[t]he annual loss of life by smallpox in the metropolis before vaccination was established exceeded 5,000'; in 1839: '[f]ormerly 5,000 died annually by small-pox in the London Bills' (the phrase being used here to denote the geographical area rather than the published documents). The bills themselves were prone to various errors of a kind typified long after their demise by a distinguished statistician who, in 1882, discussing the power of vaccination as a preventive of smallpox, asserted that there could be no answer 'except such as is couched in the language of figures', and proceeded to draw inferences from mortality rates in the same localities at different periods taking no account of factors such as changes in population figures, the ages of victims and the conditions of their daily lives.[5]

Whatever their shortcomings the bills were and remain the only regular source of information available to students of death from smallpox during more than two centuries, and opinions of their value have varied. Creighton surprisingly thought them reasonably reliable for the eighteenth century, and so does Dixon. Gale sees them as 'only a very rough guide to the actual number of deaths from 1720 to 1837'. Within these limitations they throw some light on the more cautious and more lurid pronouncements about deaths from smallpox in London in the years before more accurate information was available, and they show the range to be much greater than is often assumed. Three times, all in the first two decades, the total was lower than 100 per year. Twelve times, in epidemic years, it rose above 3,000, reaching a peak of 3,992 in 1782. In forty years the figure was somewhere in the 1,000 range, in thirty it rose to over 2,000. There was a general decline in the last two decades of the century apart from a leap to 3,500 in 1781 (following on 871 in 1780), and a similar leap to 3,548 in 1796 (followed by 522 in 1797). The worst decade was 1761 to 1770 when the total in round figures reached almost a quarter of a million. According to Baxby, throughout the century there was no reduction in the severity of natural smallpox; the only endemic infectious diseases in England with higher death rates than smallpox were tuberculosis and fevers – typhus, typhoid and scarlet fever; and in 1796 the ratio of smallpox to other deaths in London was the highest of the century.

CHAPTER 5

THE SUTTONIAN SYSTEM

If the language of eighteenth-century figures is to be relied on, a surprising state of affairs is revealed. By the end of the third decade the contentious novelty inoculation had virtually died out, while the number of deaths from smallpox, as recorded in the London bills of mortality, remained at a steady level. Why had inoculation fallen out of favour? In 1749 the physician Frewen looked back over its vicissitudes during the period:

> it is wonderful with how great an expectation it was received, with how much industry it was cultivated, and how soon it became incredibly famous [...] Yet, notwithstanding, it made but a slow progress for several years, as gaining but little credit among the common sort of people, who began to dispute among themselves about the lawfulness of propagating disease and whether or no the small-pox produced by inoculation would be a certain security against taking it again by infection, and also whether other diseases or morbid contaminations of the blood might not be likely to be engrafted along with it.

These questions, Frewen commented, had been answered long ago 'to the satisfaction of men of learning and candour', but not, as he avoided saying, to that of the common sort of people, mainly because they were neither consulted nor offered the opportunity to try out the new discovery for themselves. Access to inoculation was and remained for many years the expensive privilege of the well-off, with the corollary pointed out in the early days of controversy by Isaac Massey, apothecary and uncle of the Revd Edmund, in a scornful dismissal of Jurin's conclusions concerning the relative dangers of natural smallpox and the inoculated variety. Those inoculated were, in accordance with Jurin's advice to medical practitioners, selected almost exclusively from the healthy, well-cared-for children of the upper classes, with all the implied built-in statistical bias. 'He forgets,' Massey complained, 'that the inoculated are picked lives. If that's fair: Hang fair!'

Several treatises published towards the middle of the century, when inoculation was recovering from a decade of unpopularity, showed how far in this, as in so much else, the faculty had found ways of improving on the system thought to be adequate by the old Greek women of Constantinople. The operation, in so far as it was carried out at all, had become a time-consuming and costly business. Because of the hazard of infection posed to others by those passing through inoculated smallpox, the prospective patient would normally be required to go and live for an indeterminate period in premises specially provided by the inoculator, during which time he would undergo a course of preparation intended chiefly to put him into the right state of mind and body for his ordeal. Opinions varied as to the appropriate length of time and how best to make use of it. For Burges, writing in 1744, the object was 'to bring [the habit] by a gradual transition from a state of activity to a state of rest, in which it is necessary the body should be when it receives the infection'. This, if the patient was in good health, could be done in three weeks, during which period

> [he] should be entirely disengaged from business of all kinds, and avoid all application and close attention; should not sit long to reading but endeavour to pass the time agreeably with a few friends. In the day time, when the weather is serene and mild, he may take the air and even walk a mile or two according to his strength [...] I think the whole may be included in three words, viz. temperance, quiet and cheerfulness.

Frewen, in the work already quoted, saw preparation as a somewhat sterner affair:

> Medicinal regimen of some sort before inoculation is, for the most part, necessary, though not always, and this is to be judged of with regard to age, habit of body and other circumstances of the patient. In a plethory, bleeding, vomiting etc. ought always to be recommended previous to the operation; and in a puny habit a light infusion of the bark, after a gentle vomit or purge, drank for some time, proves greatly beneficial. But in a gross or robust habit, I would always recommend a course of aethiopsmineral or cinnobar, with a milk-diet, for a month or six weeks after plentiful bleeding or purging [...] The properest of all vomiting medicines is the radix ipecaconhae...

In addition to the fortnight or so which the disease took to run its course the treatment must always provide for a suitable period of recovery before the patient could return home and resume normal life. Little wonder that the common sort of people, calculating the loss of several weeks' wages on top of the inoculator's fee, should come to the conclusion that the benefits of inoculation were not for them or their families; and even those fortunate citizens with time on their hands and money to spare might think twice before taking the plunge. But what of the possible horrifying alternative? Smallpox was notoriously no respecter of persons.

'Lord Dalkeith is dead of the smallpox in three days', Horace Walpole wrote in 1750. 'It is so dreadfully fatal in his family that, besides several uncles and aunts, his eldest boy died of it last year, and his only brother, who was ill but two days, putrefied so fast that his limbs fell off as they lifted the body into the coffin.' It was against sickening catastrophes of this kind that practitioners stressed the safety and peace of mind provided by inoculation. Frewen claimed that in his own practice, out of 300 patients between two years old and fifty, 'I have had the good fortune to meet with only one miscarriage, which would not have occurred if the preparatory requirements had been complied with'. 'Miscarriage', presumably death, may have been rare, but severe reactions to the inoculated disease, generally unrecorded, must have been frequent. There was, for example, the case of a child, described by an indignant acquaintance as 'a fine, ruddy boy, about eight years of age', who was sent away to a surgeon for a preparatory process which lasted six weeks:

> He was bled, to ascertain whether his blood was fine; was purged repeatedly, till he became emaciated and feeble; was kept on a very low diet, small in quantity, and dosed with diet drink to sweeten the blood. After this barbarism of human veterinary practice he was removed to one of the then usual inoculation stables and haltered up with others in a terrible state of disease, although none died.[1]

By good fortune the boy escaped with 'a mild exhibition of the disease', which must nevertheless have made a deep impression on him, and determined much of the course of his later life. His name was Edward Jenner.

Although the authors of treatises dealt with inoculation in terms of adult patients, it was not disputed that the highest rates of mortality from smallpox occurred among children, and for that reason some practitioners were eventually advising that the earlier a child was inoculated the better. Maty recommended parents to have the operation performed as soon as possible after the child was born. Others rejected this advice on the ground that the newborn child had enough problems to contend with while adapting to its new environment without having to take on the additional burden of a potentially hazardous disease.

'Nature,' Thomas Percival wrote,

> feeble and irritable as she then is, can scarcely struggle with the diseases to which she is ordinarily exposed [...] It is demonstrated from the bills of mortality, that two thirds of all who are born live not to be two years old, and I think it is more than probable, that a considerable proportion of these die under the age of six weeks.

Maty's proposal, therefore, 'would considerably diminish the benefits arising from inoculation and would be of dangerous and fatal consequence to mankind'. The most forcible argument against the practice of very early inoculation was the ill success it had met with, as demonstrated by the investigations of Jurin and his successor Scheuchzer: 'of fifty-eight children under two years old who received the small-pox by ingraftment, six died, whereas of two hundred and twenty one, inoculated between the ages of two and five, only three died'. By the time when Burges, Frewen and others were writing, the lesson seems largely to have sunk in: the earliest age generally settled on was two years, with a preference for getting the job done, if possible, by the time the child was five. Jenner, an orphan brought up by an elder bachelor brother in a fairly remote part of the country, was perhaps just unlucky to have had to wait for a further three years.

By the middle of the century inoculation was making steady, albeit slow progress, with the aid of demonstrations of faith by individuals and public institutions. At the Foundling Hospital, which had received its charter in 1739, the successful inoculation of fourteen three-year-olds led the governors to have all their children inoculated in future at that age. In 1746 a proposal was put forward for a hospital for the reception of persons casually infected with the smallpox, with an additional one for inoculating the poor. The project suffered the inevitable delays of its kind and although by 1750 there had been 620 cases of natural smallpox under the charity's care only 34 patients had been admitted to be inoculated, in what were still only temporary premises. When a new hospital was finally completed in 1768 the number of inoculations, which had stood at no more than 659, rose dramatically to 1,084. Of the 6,581 inoculations performed during the period from

1749 it was claimed that 'the unsuccessful [...] were in the proportion of one in 250'.

These measures were not greeted everywhere with the kind of response that the philanthropic promoters may have expected. Unlike the isolated establishments to which the upper and middle classes withdrew for their operations, the Smallpox Hospital was sited in a densely populated area of London, and the poorer classes objected strongly to what they saw as an unacceptable health hazard in their midst. The churchwardens and overseers of the poor in the parish of Clerkenwell tried to get an injunction from the Court of Chancery to prevent the trustees of the Hospital from taking in any person affected with smallpox. They failed and the building went ahead as planned, but Woodville records that the prejudices against it were so great that 'patients on leaving it were abused and insulted in the street; wherefore they were not suffered to depart until the darkness of the night enabled them to do it unobserved by the populace'.

The President of the Hospital was the Bishop of Worcester, Dr Maddox. In 1752, choosing deliberately, perhaps, the church in which Edmund Massey had preached his inflammatory sermon against inoculation thirty years earlier, Maddox delivered an equally powerful and persuasive defence.[2] His medical arguments were to some extent vitiated by an inevitable reliance on the received wisdom of the age: inoculation was 'not so properly the giving a distemper to a human body intirely free from and out of danger of that distemper, as choosing the safest time and manner of causing a disorder, otherwise almost unavoidable in a way extremely more pernicious, the fuel thereof being lodged within us'; a reference to the current doctrine of the 'morbid seed' of smallpox which would at some time ripen into the externally visible and possibly mortal disease. Inoculation must always be 'pursued with the utmost care and precaution', but there could be no religious objection to it, even though it might not be 'universally successful', as the Bishop demonstrated in an implicit and dignified rebuttal of Massey's inane ramblings on the fate of Job:

> in order to excite and secure a dependence upon his divine providence, the Great Governor of the world has appointed that no human affairs, not even our necessary sustenance, should be attended with such absolute certainty: a very wise appointment! that vain man might not fancy himself an independent being; but among all the changes and chances of this mortal life, should still look up unto, because he can only be defended by, God's most gracious and ready help.

Inoculation was still something of a lottery but the faithful could rest assured that the wheel was at least spun by an almighty and beneficent hand.

So, with the mandatory appeal to the evidence of the bills of mortality (which showed smallpox raging that year with unparalleled fury, reaching a total of more than 3,500 deaths) and a passing reference to 'this unhappy period, when debauchery and vice, with the most destructive and as it were pestilential intemperance are making dreadful havock among the inhabitants of this island', the Bishop commended the Smallpox Hospital to the charitable impulses of his well-heeled congregation.

Inoculation was now spreading gradually over the whole kingdom, and was given a welcome boost when, in 1754, a significant branch of the medical profession took a decisive step forward. The College of Physicians,

> having been informed, that false reports concerning the success of inoculation in England, have been published in foreign countries, think proper to declare their sentiments in the following manner; viz. That the arguments which at the commencement of this practice were urged against it, have been refuted by experience; that it is now held by the English in greater esteem and practised among them more extensively than ever it was before; and that the College thinks it to be highly salutary to the human race.[3]

The principal obstacle to the wider extension of inoculation to the mass of the population, apart from its general unpopularity, remained the costly and cumbersome procedures insisted on by the medical profession. Even at the Smallpox and Inoculation Hospitals, where the treatment was free, a commentator noted that 'persons who availed themselves of it were obliged to submit to the inconvenience of two months' confinement at considerable expense to the charity'. Clearly a new broom was needed, and in the 1760s it arrived and changed the scene irrevocably.

If a specific event could be said to have inaugurated the new era it would be the occasion sometime in the late 1730s when the eldest son of a surgeon, having been inoculated by one of his father's colleagues, developed smallpox and nearly died. This inspired the parent, Robert Sutton, to look for a less perilous way of carrying out the operation. By 1755 he had pursued his research sufficiently far to attempt a trial inoculation and two years later to advertise that he had taken a commodious house and was ready to receive patients who were 'disposed to be inoculated for the small-pox'. By 1762 he was employing his new system with steadily increasing success. The practice prospered and expanded in step with the size of his family, until the day arrived when six of his sons had followed in their father's footsteps and were employing his method, or perhaps their own variation of it, over a large part of England and even on the Continent.

The system was developed to its greatest extent by Robert's second son, Daniel, whose fame soon eclipsed that of his father. His impact from the time when he set up his own practice in 1763 was unparalleled in the medical world, and he himself came to embody much of the spirit of the age, a typical product of the Industrial Revolution and a worthy contemporary, in his own line, of its better known figures.

In the last quarter of the eighteenth century the population of England and Wales rose to nine million, three quarters of them still living in rural areas, many still farming the land, but far more working in village industries which had not yet been sucked dry to swell the workforce of the exploding industrial cities. A generation of inventors and entrepreneurs was emerging and laying the foundations of a new social and economic landscape, in which the firm of Sutton, exploiting their new inoculation system, had their own part to play. In 1767 Watt patented his steam engine and Hargreaves began the transformation of the cotton industry with his spinning jenny. Crompton's mule dates from 1775. These were merely the advance guard of the army of innovators. According to G. M. Trevelyan, 'The patents issued in the quarter of a century following 1760 were more numerous than those issued in the previous century and a half'.[4] Mass production and improved marketing techniques were similarly making great strides. For example, 'Between 1760 and 1790 [Wedgwood] succeeded in filling not only England but Europe and America with his goods'. In remarkably similar words James Moore, two hundred years ago, described how Daniel Sutton 'with secret nostrums, propagated inoculation more in half a dozen years than both the Faculties of Medicine and Surgery with the aid of the church and the example of the court had been able to do in half a century'. Where the Frewens and Burgeses and their kind, catering for their leisured class of patrons, counted their inoculations in hundreds over decades, Daniel Sutton, established in his practice at Ingatestone, near Chelmsford, was soon counting his in thousands: in 1764, 1,629; in 1765, 4,347; in 1766, 7,816; a total of 13,792, not including the operations, amounting to at least 6,000, performed by assistants. Clarkson records that 'by 1776 Sutton and his associates claimed to have inoculated 300,000 people, many of them paupers treated free of charge'.

The inoculation business as a whole flourished at this period in rural areas and country towns, as many advertisements in local newspapers show. The operators were often no more than apothecaries offering a service alongside their normal business of dispensing medicines. There had previously been little hard selling, let alone cut-throat competition, in the profession; whatever their other faults, and allowing for a certain amount of peevish jousting by pamphlet, medical practitioners had been willing, as their publications indicate, to share their knowledge and expertise with each other and the public. Daniel Sutton soon changed all that. He couldn't patent his own or his father's discoveries, but he could take refuge in a policy known to later generations as 'commercial confidentiality', in other words, keeping his secrets as far as possible from prying eyes, while at the same time stimulating public curiosity and demand with the aid of an advertising executive or public relations consultant. The fact that this employee was a minister of religion, describing himself as 'officiating clergyman' on a salary of £200 a year, at the chapel provided by Sutton for the spiritual welfare of his patients appears to have disconcerted neither man, and allowed Sutton to cast the net of his own gospel more widely and stridently than the more staid members of the faculty would have thought acceptable.

In 1766 the Revd Robert Houlton in his dual capacity preached at Ingatestone a sermon in defence of inoculation, on the text 'This sickness is not unto death' (John 11.4). He took the debate about inoculation into new territory by introducing the notion of guilt on the part of parents, which subsequently became a favourite tactic among inoculators and even more among vaccinators. The published version of the sermon was prefaced by an address to Sutton which left little doubt as to the working relationship between the two men:

> Your indefatigable attention to investigate the true and abstruse nature of the small-pox, the surprisingly great improvements you have made in the practice of inoculation, have rendered it a blessing indeed; and merited you the distinguished favour and applause of the public. By these improvements the art justly becomes your own, an art that must and ought to transmit your name to posterity. And it is not to be doubted, but the time is hastily approaching, when the SUTTONIAN system or method of inoculation will be universally adopted.
>
> Here, sir, I seem to see the odious, ghostly sneers of the unskilful, the envious and ill-affected. But let me tell the wretches, they have no right to question the above truths, or to stigmatise

me with the name of flatterer, until they have proved themselves superior to you in experience, practice and success.

Picking up the thread of the earlier preacher, Bishop Maddox, who had attempted to re-define the position of God in relation to inoculation, Houlton now re-defined the parent in relation to God in this context, giving it an emphasis that came to dominate controversy on the theme for more than a century.

The key word was 'sin'. Inoculation represented the most complete victory over the dreadful enemy smallpox, and therefore a triumph over death. 'Not to make a proper use of this blessing is to sin against knowledge, to rebel against light, to act against reason and to disregard experience, the best of wisdom.' The purpose of inoculation was to lengthen and preserve life; but

> can we say we are strictly satisfied in our conscience that we are pleasing to God, by neglecting to use those salutary means for the preservation of life which have long been practised with his blessing? [...] It is reasonable to suppose, if the Almighty was displeased with the action, he would have long ago shown marks of his displeasure.

He had not done so, and 'because the intention is good the practice of inoculation can be justified in the sight of God and ourselves'.

Having dealt with religious objections, Houlton next addressed the scruples and fears of conscientious parents, who might never forgive themselves if their children should die as a result of the operation.

> In the first place we answer, there is scarce a possibility of death attending the action, so safe is the practice and so great is the perfection to which it is now brought. But allowing that some infants may die, no sin is incurred, because the act is not forbidden, and our intention [...] is to do good, to save life, not to destroy it.

But the best reply to make to all scrupulous parents was to ask them:

> If you neglect to have your children inoculated, and they are infected, as they grow up, with the natural small-pox and die, have you not real cause to be uneasy, and to accuse yourselves of carelessness and want of natural affection, as the means to have saved their lives, at least from this kind of death, were so manifestly efficacious and so indisputably safe?

The question is still being asked today in similar contexts.

In the following year William Watson, FRS, FRCP and a trustee of the British Museum, published his own short treatise *On the most successful method of inoculating the small-pox*. Naming no names he cast a different light on Houlton's assurances:

Within these last ten years [i.e. from 1758 to 1768] there have died within the compass of the bills of mortality only, twenty-three thousand three hundred and eight persons [...] Of these, how many died under inoculation we are not informed. It were a desirable thing to be known [...] The deaths by inoculation ought to make a distinct article in the bills of mortality. In great numbers inoculated some will die, whoever may conduct the process: but as many inoculators endeavour industriously to conceal the deaths in this practice, and are desirous of attributing them to any cause rather than the small-pox, it would not be easy to procure the real numbers.

Forty years later, when vaccination had largely supplanted inoculation, James Moore, an ardent advocate of the former and opponent of the latter, took an even stronger line:

An exact calculation cannot [...] be made of the proportion of deaths among those who were inoculated and skilfully treated: because the interest and vanity of medical men prompt them to exaggerate their success, and to conceal their failures: even the reports of hospitals cannot be relied on: for the parents of the inoc-ulated, from discontent, from grief, or from residing at a distance, sometimes neglect to give information when their children are dangerously attacked, and when they perish.[5]

Not content with dismissing the religious and conscientious scruples of parents, Houlton even ventured into the realm of politics:

What inestimable advantages do the public reap from inoculation! [...] If every child's life is of great value to the community, of how much more consequence are the lives of lusty youths and robust men! All, all are saved by inoculation: but thousands, thro' neglect of it, are every year cut off in the prime of youth and manhood.

The inference was plain: it was up to the Government to do all in its power to promote inoculation, 'and more especially at this time when the nation is so thin of men, that it is well known, and severely felt, thousands are wanted among the lower class, to perform the common works of husbandry and labour. But how would this scarcity of people be felt, if we were to be engaged soon again in another war!'

In an appendix to his published sermon Sutton's officiating clergyman let himself go with an encomium which recalled that golden age on the shores of the Bosphorus when being engrafted in the Greek fashion was such fun:

> The slightness of [Mr Sutton's] operation in communicating the infection [...] is easier than one can possibly conceive. With respect to pain, it is not equal to the thousandth part which the prick of a pin gives. The operation is performed on most without their knowing it: and in a minute afterwards the puncture is scarce visible [...] The patients in general have little or no sickness: their indisposition is so trifling that they are ashamed to complain, and in a few days they are perfectly well. There is no confinement, no keeping of bed. All is mirth and all are happy. In fact this fortnight's visit to Mr Sutton's abounds with real pleasure and satisfaction. The pleasing conversation of the company, added to their various amusements, makes the time glide away imperceptibly.

* * *

What was the reality behind this façade? The foundation was the simplified technique of inoculating which was pioneered by Robert Sutton and consisted of taking matter from a donor at an earlier stage in the development of a smallpox vesicle than had previously been the practice: this was then introduced into the arm of the recipient in a manner described by Daniel Sutton in his book *The Inoculator*: 'The lancet being charged with the smallest possible quantity (and the smaller the better) of unripe, crude or watery matter, introduce it by puncture obliquely, between the scarf and the skin, barely sufficient to draw blood and not deeper than the sixteenth part of an inch'. To achieve this the blade of the lancet would lie almost flat in contact with the arm, in contrast to the heavy-handed incisions favoured by Nettleton and others among the early operators.

This procedure, preceded by a modified preparatory 'regimen' and followed by the cool and relaxing regimen of recovery described by Houlton, imposed on the patient a less taxing burden and in the long run helped to lower the mortality rate, although whether to the extent claimed by practitioners has been questioned. Chandler, one of a number of physicians and surgeons who, in 1767, published pamphlets speculating and disagreeing with each other as to the precise elements of the Suttonian system, paid the promoter of it a slightly back-handed compliment:

> It ought to be observed, in justice to Mr Sutton that every part of his practice in inoculation carries with it strong marks of solid judgment and accurate observation. Considering that he has to all appearances borrowed many hints from authors which are in everybody's hands, it is a matter of some surprise that this many parts of his practice have not before been generally adopted by others.

Some years later Moore accepted that Daniel's plan of treatment was 'greatly superior' to that of any former practitioner, but concluded that as far as their medicines were concerned 'the Suttons in strictness invented nothing: but judiciously combined remedies which had been found out independently by others'. Daniel's success 'though exaggerated was great', but the secrets of his success could not be maintained for long because so many thousands of patients and knowledgeable rivals soon acquired a first-hand acquaintance with the details.

One critic of the system maintained, along with the occasional disgruntled client, that it sometimes produced so little visible effect that what had been communicated, whatever else it might have been, was not smallpox, and the recipient had therefore been defrauded; but this was not the popular view. The Suttonian system swept the board, making its promoters rich, and became the unchallenged method for decades until inoculation as a preventive against smallpox was banned by Parliament in 1840, by which time it had been superseded by vaccination. Yet although Sutton gave his name to the system, he published no account of his methods until 1796, by which time his personal fame had for long been overtaken by that of a surgeon whose treatise on inoculation, first published in 1767, and running through many editions, became the standard textbook on the subject, and he himself one of its most illustrious and prosperous exponents.

Thomas Dimsdale, a Quaker from an old-established Essex family, began practising as a surgeon in Hertford, retired when his second marriage made him a wealthy man but not sufficiently so to sustain a rather extravagant lifestyle, and returned to the profession, this time as a physician, in 1761, shortly before the appearance on the national scene of Daniel Sutton. It has been suggested that Dimsdale may have acted briefly as Sutton's assistant, which, if true, would account for his

early mastery of the Suttonian system. His own practice expanded
rapidly, largely because, in the words of one biographer, 'he was a
polished man of the world, his methods of acquiring practice were
orthodox and... he inspired confidence in people who wanted the
Suttonian technique but shied at [Sutton's] rough manners and the
rowdy way he permitted his patients to behave while under his care'.

In so far as so successful a man needed a lucky break Dimsdale's may
be said to have arrived in 1768. Catherine the Great of Russia,
throughout whose vast realm smallpox was endemic and uncontrolled,
had come to the conclusion that the solution to her problem lay in the
introduction of a reputable form of inoculation. She sought a reliable
practitioner from England, as the source of the latest methods, to travel
to Russia and set the ball rolling for her. Another of the rumours that
attach themselves to Daniel Sutton suggests that he was nominated as
the first choice but that he declined, not liking the sound of the
proposal, which was then passed to Dimsdale, who accepted it and set
off in July 1768, accompanied by one of his sons, for St Petersburg.
There is some reason to believe that he was unaware until he arrived
that his first patient was not to be, as he had supposed, the Grand
Duke, the heir to the throne, but the Empress herself who, although
the details of the operation would be kept secret until it was over,
wanted to be seen to have set a good example to her people. The implications for Dimsdale were underlined for him by the court official to
whom he reported:

> You are now called, sir, to the most important employment that
> perhaps any gentleman was ever entrusted with. To your skill and
> integrity will [...] be submitted no less than the precious lives of
> two of the greatest personages in the world, with whose safety the
> tranquillity and happiness of this great empire are so intimately
> connected that should an accident deprive us of either, the bless-
> ings we now enjoy might be turned to the utmost state of misery
> and confusion. May God avert such unspeakable calamities.[6]

Whether or not these were the precise words used they no doubt
summed up the situation accurately. Dimsdale later learnt that relays of
post horses had been standing by to get him and his son with all
possible speed from St Petersburg to the Russian border in the event of
a mishap.

Fortunately they had no need to make an ignominious retreat by the
back door: on the contrary, both operations were carried out with
conspicuous success (after a brief delay while the Grand Duke

contracted and recovered from chickenpox), and a grateful Empress paid Dimsdale £10,000, with a pension of £500 a year, made him a baron and enabled him to style himself 'Physician and Actual Counseller of State to her Imperial Majesty the Empress of all the Russias' – a royal warrant, if it wasn't self-conferred, more resounding than anything he might have picked up in his native land. The honour conferred carried obligations that were not always welcome: the Empress was apt to summon him for advice, medication or just tea and sympathy on comparatively trivial pretexts, keeping him on call in Russia when he would have preferred to be back home. This may explain why some of his major works were written and first published in St Petersburg, appearing only some years later in England.

By Dimsdale's day a good deal of the rigmarole surrounding the process of inoculation had been stripped away. For example:

> I remember a time when the inoculator thought it necessary to use every precaution that could be suggested to prevent the supposed danger of communicating the natural disease. The patient's head was turned aside, a handkerchief sprinkled with spirits of lavender water, or some volatile spirit, was held to the nose and the inoculator was as expeditious as possible in performing the operation, making afterwards a precipitous retreat, as if he were an assassin.[7]

Or again, from an account of the Smallpox Hospital:

> Experience assures us that a person who is in good health may be safely inoculated without any preparation, and that all regulations in respect to diet and the necessary course of medicine may be sufficiently complied with in the week that intervenes between the operation and the commencement of the disease.[8]

As to the post-operative regime,

> Those who have the disease [...] without any appearance of eruption but on the inoculated part are soon allowed to go about their usual affairs; and many instances have happened of poor men [...] who have instantly returned to their daily labours, with a caution not to intermix with those who have not had the distemper, for fear of spreading it.[9]

At the end of his exposition of inoculation as it was performed at this time Dimsdale asked to what particular circumstances its success was owing, and concluded that 'perhaps we should be found to have improved but little upon the judicious Sydenham's cool method of treating the disease, and the old Greek woman's method of inoculating with fluid matter carried warm in her servant's bosom'.[10]

In sharp contrast to the operation performed on individual patients, in the simplified version popularized by Sutton, Dimsdale and others, was the growth of mass inoculation, which seemed to run counter to one of the basic principles of treatment (somewhat cursorily dismissed in the passage from Dimsdale quoted above) that had been standard ever since Maitland's discovery that the inoculated disease was as infectious, and therefore potentially as lethal, as the casual kind. This, as Moore commented, had been 'a circumstance totally unexpected and it ought to have induced the profession to pause e'er they proceeded, or at least to have prompted them never to inoculate without adequate measures being adopted to prevent infection spreading to others'.

The reasons that led to neglect of this elementary precaution may have been various: in some cases incompetence, in others greed (although the beneficiaries were quite likely to be the poor, who were getting their jabs free), and most probable of all a conviction that, if properly handled, inoculation offered the possibility of 'exterminating' or 'extirpating' smallpox, one of the greatest scourges known to human-kind. The logic of this argument appeared unanswerable. If everyone were to be inoculated at the same time no one could catch the disease from anyone else, because you could only have it once, whether casually or artificially: hence the pressure in some quarters, resisted strenuously in others, for children, the chief victims of smallpox throughout the eighteenth century, to be inoculated as early in life as possible. As the years passed and the battle against the disease seemed to be progressing too slowly, or even to be in danger of being lost, a certain impatience appears to have taken over. Inoculating people, mainly the well-off, in penny numbers was doing nothing for the poor: let them therefore be treated en masse, gratis if necessary, until smallpox was starved out of existence for want of bodies to feed on.

According to Downie it was Dimsdale who introduced mass inocula-tion, but not surprisingly Daniel Sutton was one of the earliest in the field. It was in 1764, shortly after his arrival in Ingatestone, that he accepted a commission to inoculate virtually the whole population, 70 of 'the better class' and more than 400 of the poor, of the village of Maldon, a few miles away. The undertaking was a success – no one died and within three weeks smallpox, which had threatened to develop into an epidemic, was said to have disappeared from the village

– but the event had wider repercussions. A year later, Chelmsford, a busy market town and regular stopping place for stage coaches on the main road from London to Colchester, Ipswich, Norwich, Harwich and so on, was visited by smallpox, with the loss of many lives. Although, as Houlton indignantly pointed out, 'every apothecary in the town was an inoculator', some of the leading citizens decided that Sutton was 'the man that inflicted Chelmsford with the small-pox, and prepared an iditement against him at the summer assizes, for a nuisance'. The Grand Jury found in his favour. The episode can have done him no harm, and led to numerous engagements to carry out similar mass inoculations. The details of one of them, as Sutton himself described them, strain credulity to the limit:

> About ten or fifteen years after I had introduced and established the new method of inoculation I was employed to inoculate a large party [...] consisting of about 700 persons. About one half of them were inoculated before twelve o'clock and the other half were begun upon at half past three in the afternoon. They were all inoculated by my own hand, from the same individual throughout [...] the medicines were procured from the same druggist...[11]

Sutton's account appears to have been accepted without comment ever since it was made, yet the more closely this Stakhanovite performance is examined the more questions seem to be begged. For example: if, to simplify the calculation, it is assumed that Sutton inoculated 720 persons, of all ages, and took a maximum, or for that matter a minimum, of twelve hours to complete the task – say, six in the morning to six in the afternoon – he would have had to deal with 60 patients every hour, or one a minute. Assuming that 'inoculated by my own hand' is to be taken literally, and that all other work, for example charging the lancets, was performed by assistants, how, even so, could one operator maintain a high standard of accuracy throughout such a long and punishing schedule? The poor were getting their inoculation free of charge, but what degree of protection were they being given and what would be the likely consequences when the 700 infected with smallpox returned to their homes? Sutton's defence would presumably have been that since all were infected at the same time they could by definition not infect each other; but the further implication that, like the inhabitants of Eyam during the outbreak of plague in 1665–66, they cut themselves off from all contact with neighbouring communities until the infection was over is too improbable to be entertained.

Sutton claimed that as his practice grew he often inoculated 'large parties to the number of from one to six or seven hundred [...] in a day', and it is hardly surprising, though scarcely commendable, that he should have felt obliged to add (perhaps with his private practice in mind as well) that 'it was not to be supposed, however generally nice in my observations, that I could pay sufficient attention to remark with precision and to determine positively in every case, or indeed in any one in particular, at the instant'.

Dimsdale, whether or not the first in the field, was an advocate of the benefits of mass inoculations, having taken part in several himself in various parishes in the neighbourhood of Hertford, his home town, and on three occasions in the town itself, the last in 1774: 'From that time we have heard nothing of small-pox and I verily believe that within these ten years not six persons have died in Hertford of the disease.' The conclusion was inescapable: the general inoculations had left hardly anyone susceptible of the disease:

> Does it not strike one obviously that, whether inoculation or the natural distemper has been so general that most of the inhabitants have undergone it, the case will be exactly the same. The place will be secure from an epidemic until a fresh race of new born children, or a change of inhabitancy has furnished the town with more subjects for the disease.[12]

There was one important proviso: mass or general inoculations must be confined for the most part to rural areas and small towns, with populations of manageable size. The larger the town or city the less possibility of the necessary precautions being observed; and at the end of the road lay the most intractable problem of all – the metropolis. In all discussions concerning the control of smallpox it was universally recognized that London was *sui generis*, a vast, overcrowded, relentlessly expanding 'great Wen', as Cobbett subsequently called it, where smallpox was endemic, with an average of 12,000 cases a year, mostly among infants and young children, and where measures that might afford protection elsewhere would be hopelessly inadequate.

While he was still in St Petersburg in 1768 or 1769, Dimsdale had written, possibly for the benefit of his Russian colleagues, a short essay under the title *Thoughts on General and Partial Inoculation*, drawing on experience gained in Britain. From a study of the bills of mortality over a period of thirty-two years and a comparison with Jurin's earlier statistics, Dimsdale found that in general, 'the small-pox carried off the eighth part of those who died in London in the period'. It was well known that 'what passes previous to the eruptive fever' could be ignored, 'since no infection can be communicated before that time'. The danger began later, when 'the disease may be spread by the inter-course of visitors, trades people, servants and others and, in a mild state of the disease, the frequent excursions of the sick by way of airings and often in carriages of various kinds contribute greatly towards spreading the infection'.[13] Whoever took the disease from an inoculated patient had the natural smallpox.

This essay, published in Russia, is unlikely to have been known in England in 1775 when a group of philanthropists, distressed by the thought that the benefits of inoculation were not widely available to the poor of London, and undaunted by the difficulties to be overcome, founded a Society for Inoculation at the Homes of the People. Dimsdale, appalled by the risks being undertaken, rushed out a translation of his essay in the hope of dissuading the philanthropists; they refused to be side-tracked, and a war of pamphlets ensued. One of Dimsdale's opponents, the physician John Lettsom, issued proposals for a *General Inoculation Dispensary for the benefit of the poor throughout London… without removing them from their homes*. Dimsdale took up the challenge again in 1778 with *Observations on the Introduction to the Plan of a Dispensary for General Inoculation*, which reiterated his arguments against the whole concept:

> those who have the disease badly will infect the cloaths, furniture or any other substances that are near them. And among the poor of London, whose situation in life neither admits of a change of raiment, or furniture, nor even the leisure necessary to clean them, the consequence of one having the small-pox very full must necessarily be that the apartment and all that is in it will remain in an infected state, and in some distant period […] the seeds of infection […] may become active and the disease will appear again.[14]

The controversy dragged on through a series of polemical salvos before petering out.

Meanwhile two hundred miles to the north-west of London another of the eighteenth century's most distinguished medical practitioners was exploring a different approach to the ravages of smallpox. John Haygarth was born in 1740 in that high part of the Yorkshire dales that borders on the Lancashire Pennines, and after attending the grammar school in Sedbergh went on to St John's College, Cambridge. He gained the degree of Bachelor of Medicine in 1766 and in due course moved to Chester where he worked for more than thirty years investigating the nature of fever and smallpox. His *Observations on the Population and Diseases of Chester* were published in the *Philosophical Transactions* of the Royal Society in 1778.

A former Roman city of great importance, Chester retains many features of its classical and mediaeval past. Until the River Dee changed its course and its estuary became silted up Chester was a flourishing port, its indigenous population constantly augmented by the passage of travellers to and from Ireland and further afield. As Haygarth depicted it, Chester was a city of more than usually striking contrasts: on the one hand, 'healthy in such an uncommon degree as will astonish those who are best acquainted with the general state of mortality in large towns'. Perched on 'a red, sandy, mouldering rock', encircled by ancient Roman walls, with its centre marking, as it still does, the intersection of the main thoroughfares of the original Roman encampment, its air was uncommonly clear; the River Dee, still tidal and navigable in the eighteenth century, flowed right up to, and at the period of spring tides into, the town, washing away 'the liquid filth' of the higher localities; the famous Rows, or covered galleries, were always dry and clean, even in wet and dirty weather, tempting abroad 'persons of a delicate and valetudinary constitution'. The inhabitants of this part of Chester had 'near an equal chance of living to twice the age of the inhabitants of Vienna, London or Edinburgh'.

On the other hand there were the suburbs, where 'a part of the putrid filth' that flowed from the centre 'stagnated in the ditches'. The dwellers in these areas were in general 'of the lowest rank; they want most of the conveniences and comforts of life: their houses are small, close, crowded and dirty: their diet affords very poor nourishment, and their cloaths are very seldom changed or washed [...] The air they breathe at home is rendered noxious by perspiration and putrefaction.' It was amid scenes of this kind that Haygarth laboured to ameliorate the conditions that caused so much suffering and death. Among his most far-reaching innovations was the provision of special wards in the infirmary in which patients suffering from contagious fevers could be isolated until they were no longer a danger to others. Besides medical treatment they were to enjoy 'clean linen, careful attendance and wholesome diet'. A modern authority has written that Haygarth's strict rules for the running of his two fever wards would, with one or two improvements, serve isolation wards today.

Haygarth's other major interest, which conditions in Chester afforded him plenty of opportunity to pursue, was the study of smallpox and how to prevent it from spreading. As with the fever wards, the key was isolation:

I argue that the variolous poison, in the form of serum, pus and scab, by impregnating the air near it, is the sole means of infection [...] The air is rendered infectious but to a little distance from the variolous poison, [which] in a house is not infectious to anyone outside it [...] One visitor in 10 or 20 may possibly convey out of an infectious room some of the variolous matter capable of doing mischief: It may accidentally adhere to some part of his cloths or person. But cleanliness alone [...] would be sufficient to prevent the communication of infection, except by personal intercourse with the patient.[15]

The sufferings of the poor during a particularly severe epidemic of smallpox in Chester in 1774 made such a deep impression on him that it became 'an object of my most anxious wishes to preserve their lives by inoculation', and in 1777, following a further epidemic, he published an *Inquiry How to Prevent the Small-pox*, and proposed the foundation of a 'Society for Promoting General Inoculation at Stated Periods and preventing the Natural Small-pox in Chester'. The first of these, which did not take place until 1780 and then in circumstances far removed from the unruly jamborees favoured by Sutton, produced less than satisfactory results.

In an attempt to overcome some of the spirit of fatalism inherent in the attitude of the poorer classes to smallpox, especially among their children, he insisted (contrary to his statements elsewhere) that humankind was not necessarily subject to the disease – it was always caught by infection 'from a patient in the distemper' and could be avoided by scrupulous observance of a set of Rules of Prevention, which although simple were as stringent as those that applied in the fever wards, relying on the same principle of isolation. No one who had not had the smallpox was to go into an infectious house, and no patient should be allowed to go into the street or other frequented places after the pocks had appeared:

The utmost attention to cleanliness is absolutely necessary; during and after the distemper no person, clothes, food, furniture, dog or cat, money, medicines or any other thing that is known or suspected to be daubed with matter, spittle or other infectious discharges of the patient should go out of the house until they have been washed...[16]

The observance of these rules, Haygarth insisted somewhat disingenuously, required little trouble and no expense, but might be 'attended with some inconvenience, especially to the poor'; so as a recompense and motive for obedience some reward should be offered on terms set out in a 'promissory note', which guaranteed a small payment by the society to a family as soon as all the scabs had 'dropt off' its infected members, on condition that the rules had been 'exactly observed', and the patients would allow a member or official of the society to inspect them. There would also be 'a reward if no neighbour or acquaintance be attacked by the small-pox during the time it is in the family… nor within 16 days after all the scabs have entirely fallen off the family'. Among the functions of the Society's inspector would be to obtain information, hand out copies of the rules and 'keep an exact register on a plan that may include every necessary information that can be required to investigate the progress of a distemper thro' a town'.

Neither the sensible steps provided for in the rules nor the financial incentive to comply with them proved sufficient to ensure the success of the scheme, as Haygarth admitted in 1792 in a letter to the Syndick and Council of the City and Republic of Geneva:

> The proceedings of the Small-pox Society of Chester were suspended soon after my former publication [presumably the *Inquiry*] was sent to the press. This suspension was occasioned neither by a medical difficulty, nor by a deficiency in the voluntary subscriptions but solely by the ignorance and delusions of the populace. Our plan was to propose gratuitous inoculation to the children of the poor of our fellow citizens every second year. At the close of the third year, when this favour was humanely offered to them it was universally rejected […] not one, or but one child could be found, whose parents would accept the intended kindness. This vulgar folly was unaccountable; for the general inoculation had been very successful, the proportional fatality not being greater than *one* in *two hundred* […] I repeat a mother's answer: 'Four of my children have already died of the common small-pox, and, if my only remaining child should die by inoculation, I could never forgive myself'.[17]

This, Haygarth commented contemptuously, was 'contrary to commonsense'.[18]

This experience may have saddened but did nothing to discourage him, merely directing his thinking into more uncompromising channels. What the poor would not accept as a gift must be forced on them by other means: or, as he expressed it, anticipating the decision of Parliament some sixty years later, '[w]hat is commonly done through a principle of benevolence and humanity the law might require to be universally performed'.[19]

This revolutionary opinion occurs towards the end of his final treatise on smallpox, *A Sketch of a plan to exterminate the casual small-pox from Great Britain and to introduce general inoculation...*, published in 1793 as a sequel to the *Inquiry*. A dedication to the King (George the Third) laments that 'so small a proportion of Your Majesty's subjects even yet enjoy the benefits of inoculation [which] is still so far confined to the superior and least numerous classes of society [and] continues to be the most fatal malady that ever afflicted mankind'. The preface suggests that the author is more than a little anxious concerning the nature of what he is about to propose:

> I must particularly entreat the reader not to pronounce a summary condemnation upon the SKETCH, nor to blacken its character by any of those harsh and discouraging expressions which all novelty upon important subjects is too apt to occasion, as, 'a visionary scheme'; 'an extravagant and dangerous innovation'; 'an invasion of personal liberty'; 'an expensive project'.[20]

The essence of the plan was a proposal for dealing with the recalcitrant poor by means of a national bureaucracy of a kind not seriously attempted as an instrument of coercion until Edwin Chadwick and Nassau Senior got to work forty years later on the New Poor Law. The basis remained the 'Rules of Prevention' as set out in the *Inquiry*, and the granting of a reward at rates to be determined by the Justice of the Peace 'for their punctual and successful observance [...] during the whole period that the patient remains in an infectious state'. This applied only to the poor: 'to such persons as require no pecuniary award public thanks to be given either in the parish church or a neighbouring newspaper...'

So much for the carrot; as for the stick:

> That a transgression of the rules be punished by a fine of £10 or £50 or £... [*sic*]; one half [going] to the informer and the other to the fund which supplies the expense of rewards. That the crime be published in the nearest newspaper. That the offender who cannot pay the fine be exposed in the nearest market town, for an hour, with the label on his breast:

> 'Behold a villain who has wilfully and wickedly spread the poison of the small-pox.'[21]

Local amateur initiative having failed, Haygarth proposed a formal legal structure based on a vast expansion of the role of the inspector as defined by the defunct Society. Britain would be divided into 500 districts of roughly equal size – about 100 square miles. To each district a surgeon or apothecary would be appointed as inspector, to live as nearly as possible in the middle, pay daily visits to all infected families in his area, see that the regulations were 'exactly observed' and keep a register of all cases of smallpox. For every ten inspectors a Director would be installed to whom they would report. The whole system would be superintended by a Commission of five physicians in London and three in Edinburgh to be appointed by His Majesty or the College of Physicians.

As it was only to be expected that 'the visits of a stranger would in some cases be disagreeable' any person would have the privilege to 'recommend a reputable surgeon or apothecary to the Director of the circuit as inspector at his own family'. For this service the family would of course be expected to pay an extra charge. Those who could not afford it would, as usual, put up with what they got. If the salary of an inspector were fixed at £56 and that of a Director at £112 per year, the cost of the establishment in England would be 32,000 guineas. The Commissioners would presumably give their services free of charge.

Haygarth clearly foresaw objections to his scheme but dismissed them with the impatience of the humanitarian passionately intent on doing good on his own terms. Without rewards for obedience and the strictest supervision 'error and prejudice will long and fatally operate against improvements, which require so many innovations in the domestick concerns and social intercourse of mankind'. An 'interesting question' was whether the medical profession would accept the proposals but, ever the optimist, Haygarth was sure that '[t]heir humane feelings would be highly gratified in being the means, under Providence, of saving the lives of a large proportion of the young generation'. It is a measure of the authoritarian fantasy-world in which even so great a physician, as Haygarth undoubtedly was, may some-times dwell that in spite of the ignominious failure of the 'Society for General Inoculation' in the face of public apathy and intransigence he could still assert his belief that 'if all concerned, both officers and people, would perform their duty exactly, the small-pox might be exterminated out of the island in a few weeks'.

The truth was that inoculation, the foundation of the whole edifice, was falling into disfavour in some quarters for a reason that was more and more openly conceded: so far from reducing the incidence of small-pox it appeared to be increasing it, often, it was said, starting epidemics where they might otherwise not have broken out. Blane, relying on widely quoted statistics, told a parliamentary committee in 1802:

> according to the London bills of mortality, for the last thirty years of the late [i.e. eighteenth] century, on an average ninety-five persons died by the small-pox out of each thousand reported in the bills. By a similar calculation there died in the first thirty years of the late century seventy only in each thousand... it appears that the mortality from the small-pox is now at an average nearly one tenth of the total mortality, and that the mortality of the small-pox has increased since the introduction of inoculation. This probably holds true to a still greater degree in the country: for before the introduction of inoculation there were certain districts in which the small-pox was unknown for twenty, thirty or forty years; so that great numbers lived and died without ever having had the small-pox.[22]

This is an admission that conflicts with the oft-repeated assurance that 'every one would have it at some time in their life'; and with the figures of 36,000 deaths bandied about by Lettsom and Blane himself. 'This is no longer the case since the dissemination of inoculation.' Blane, it should be noted, was an ardent advocate of vaccination and *ipso facto* an enemy of inoculation.

William Heberden junior, a widely respected authority, the first to distinguish between chickenpox and smallpox, and author of *A Treatise on the increase and decrease of different diseases* (1801), argued that however beneficial inoculation had proved to be to individuals, and indeed to the nation at large, one class of the population had gained little from it for reasons that were well known but less readily acknowledged:

> The poor, who have little care of preserving their lives beyond the getting of their daily bread, make a very large portion of mankind. Their prejudices are strong and not easily overcome by reason. Hence while the inoculation of the wealthy keeps up a perpetual source of infection, many others who either cannot afford or do not choose to adopt the same method are continually exposed to the distemper, and the danger is still further increased by the inconsiderate manner in which it has lately been the custom to send into the open air persons in every stage of the disease, without any regard to the safety of their neighbours.[23]

Among those whom Heberden might have had in mind were practitioners such as Dr William Buchan, author of *Domestic Medicine*, an immensely popular do-it-yourself guide published in 1769, which went through 18 editions and sold 80,000 copies. In the doctor's opinion no special skills were required for the communication of the disease:

> Common sense and prudence alone are sufficient both in the choice of the subject and management of the operation. Whoever is possessed of these may perform their office for his children whenever he finds it convenient provided they be in a good state of health [...] for several years past I have persuaded parents and nurses to perform the entire operation themselves [...] common mechanics often, to my knowledge, perform the operation with as good success as physicians.[24]

He particularly recommended the clergy to take on the job: 'Most of them know something of medicine. Almost all of them bleed and can order a purge, which are all the qualifications necessary for the practice of inoculation.' Buchan at least preached what he practised, having inoculated his own son with 'a thread which had been previously wet with fresh matter from a pock, laid upon the child's arm and covered with a piece of sticking plaster': in which state the boy was presumably sent out to join his unprotected playmates.

This lack of consideration had even been extended, as Moore recalled, to the Smallpox Hospital which, besides treating victims of the casual disease, also carried out inoculation. In its early days the inoculated had been confined to a suitable building and not discharged until they were no longer infectious. 'Unhappily the wise regulations of the humane founders of the charity were afterwards altered; when all who applied at the gates were promiscuously inoculated with small-pox and suffered to wander about diffusing far and wide the morbid infection.' Moore advocated the passing of a law that would confine the inoculated to their own houses or in a hospital set aside for the purpose until they ceased to be a source of danger: 'By such a measure the infection of the small-pox, for want of any subjects to act upon would necessarily decline and soon become extinct.' Legislation of this kind was unlikely to make much appeal to a government that, for all the evidence before its eyes, had remarkably little time or inclination to bother with the problem of smallpox.

By the 1780s, as the disease was reaching the zenith of its destructive powers, mass inoculations, as Creighton showed, were being undertaken all over the British Isles, from cities as populous as Leeds and Liverpool to villages as remote as Applecross on the coast of Ross, many of them carried out 'in so haphazard a manner as to make them value-less for a scientific as well as for a practical purpose'. His conclusion, surveying the eighteenth century in retrospect, was that

> whatever its theoretical correctness it does not follow that inocula-tion was a practical success to the extent of its trial, and that its theoretical correctness will be thought by some, and was so thought at the time, to have gone by the board when the artificial disease was brought down to a pustule at the point of a puncture with or without a few bastard pocks on the skin near.[25]

The only hope, short of the decline of smallpox from natural causes, lay in the opening up of some new way forward which would offer the benefits of inoculation with fewer of its drawbacks. At this point, in 1798, Edward Jenner stepped into the limelight, proclaiming the prophylactic power of a disease of cattle commonly referred to in agri-cultural circles as 'the cowpox'.

CHAPTER 6

THE GREAT BENEFACTOR

Edward Jenner was, until recent years, badly served by his biographers. The first choice, although to all appearances well equipped for the task, 'entered upon it' as he confessed, 'with a degree of anxiety in which I can scarcely expect any to sympathise', and predictably made rather a hash of it. John Baron, a qualified physician and surgeon, first met Jenner in 1808 when he was fifty-nine and Baron twenty-three. They became and remained close friends and Baron was possibly the last person to see Jenner alive before his death in 1823. In view of their long and intimate acquaintance there was presumably some expectation or at least hope that Baron might play Boswell to Jenner's Johnson, but nothing could have been less likely.

A practical obstacle was the amount of time and labour involved:

The papers [...] were extremely voluminous and in the greatest disorder [...] I anxiously wished and indeed had determined to relinquish my task altogether: in addition therefore to the exertion demanded by the subject itself I may be permitted to state that my professional avocations necessarily prevented me from giving that unbroken and undivided attention indispensable to the rapid progress of a work of this nature.

A more deep-seated reason for the failure of the book lay in the relationship between the two men which, because of the age difference and Baron's deference in the face of Jenner's achievement and reputation, was more like that of father and son than of professional equals, even when later in life Baron himself had arrived at considerable eminence. There was, if Baron is to be believed, no awkwardness or keeping of distance; on the contrary, recalling their first meeting Baron commented, 'I little thought that it would so speedily lead to an intimacy and ultimately to a friendship which terminated only at his death... He condescended as to an equal; the restraint and embarrassment that might naturally have been felt in the presence of one so eminent vanished in an instant.' For his part, Jenner, in one of his few known references to Baron, made a year or two after they first met, described him as 'one of the first men in point of talent the country has to boast of'. On the night his wife died in 1815 he wrote to Baron, 'I know no one whom I should like to see here better than yourself, and as often as you can find a little leisure pray come and exercise your pity'.

The problem lay in Baron's conception of the obligation owed by a biographer to his subject. Where Boswell, for example, for all his admiration and affection for Johnson, was determined to present him in the round with the scrupulous fidelity to every aspect of the man that is the hallmark of the work, Baron went to the opposite extreme; nothing but good should be written of the deceased, and that must be expressed in the most flattering terms:

Newton had unfolded the doctrine of light and colour before he was twenty, Bacon wrote his *Temporis Partis Maximus* before he attained that age; Montesquieu had sketched his *Spirit of Laws* at an equally early period of life; and Jenner, when he was still younger, contemplated the possibility of removing from among the list of human diseases one of the most mortal that ever scourged our race.[1]

Of Jenner's first successful inoculation with cowpox:

Were I to fix upon any period in the life of this admirable man that was more full than another of deep and intense emotion, more elevated by anxious and benevolent hopes, more absorbed with generous and ardent wishes for the complete success of a scheme fraught with great and disinterested benefit to his fellow men, I would mention that portion of it which we have now been contemplating. The situation in which he then stood seldom had a parallel in the history of our race...[2]

In any dispute Jenner was almost invariably on the right side and therefore in no need of defence: 'It is distressing to know that Dr. Jenner and those who thought with him could not act as became them in this emergency without having motives ascribed to them of a very unworthy nature. It cannot be required of me to attempt to vindicate Dr. Jenner from any insinuation of this kind.'[3] Of one of the many major controversies in which Jenner was involved:

It is not my wish to dwell longer on this unpleasant topic and I have abstained from printing many of the documents from which the preceding facts are drawn [...] indeed I would gladly have passed them by altogether had not the character of Dr. Jenner and still more the character of vaccination been materially affected by them.

On at least one occasion he carried this policy of total censorship into effect: details concerning the publication of Jenner's ground-breaking *Inquiry*, which are not wholly to his credit, are omitted altogether and must be searched for elsewhere. A modern authority has accused Baron in this instance of deliberately attempting to deceive.

As an account of Jenner's life and achievement, therefore, Baron's work is little more than an exercise in hagiography, but in the absence of a competing version it remained virtually unchallenged for decades, until the introduction of legislation based on Jenner's theories led to vicious assaults on his doctrines and his character, portraying the Great Benefactor as little better than the Great Impostor.

The pendulum inevitably had to swing again: aspects of his work were occasionally reassessed and he himself was rehabilitated in more moderate terms, but the only attempt at a biography of any length was unfortunately couched in a 'told-to-the-children' style ('As his quill scratched the last few lines [of his *Inquiry*] over the hand-made paper his full mouth curled into smiles and his eyes shone'), depicting him, against much of the evidence, as 'one of the most lovable gentlemen in all Gloucestershire'. It is only in recent times that a full, discerning and scholarly biography has been written by Robert Fisher, doing justice to Baron's 'admirable man'.

The present work, being concerned to trace the origins and later the course of the controversy that vaccination gave rise to, neither requires nor would justify the recapitulation of every aspect of Jenner's life. The account that follows therefore confines itself in the first instance to the broad outlines of his career and will go into greater detail in the appropriate place concerning the attacks made on him fifty years after his death.

Born in 1749 in Berkeley, a remote village in Gloucestershire, the son of the local vicar, Jenner was orphaned at the age of five – his parents died within two months of each other – and was brought up by a bachelor brother, also a vicar and some years older than himself. When he was eight he was sent to school at Wooton-under-Edge, a few miles from home, where he experienced his stressful inoculation for smallpox, and later moved to Sodbury to receive instruction in surgery and pharmacy from a local practitioner. His first big step into the wider world took him to London where he had the good fortune to spend two years as the pupil of John Hunter, the surgeon to St George's hospital, variously described as 'an anatomist and comparative zoologist' (Baxby) and 'one of the founders of experimental pathology and biology' (Greenwood), and undoubtedly one of the outstanding scientists of the day.

It was through Hunter's influence that in 1771 Jenner was given the task of preparing and arranging the specimens brought back by Sir Joseph Banks from Cook's first voyage of exploration. He apparently performed the task to everyone's satisfaction and was invited to join the next expedition as naturalist, an offer he declined. Baron's comment, hardly a sufficient explanation of the decision, is typical: 'Possibly [...] we may now be permitted to trace the agency of a higher power, which induced a young man frequently to reject the most flattering proposals of wealth and distinction that he might be enabled to follow up the leading object of his mind in the seclusion of a country village.'[4] We might, on the other hand, do better to recall the verdict of a man whose acquaintance with Jenner pre-dated that of Baron by a good many years and who contrasted Jenner's 'activity of mind' with his 'indolence of person and habits of procrastination', concluding that he 'showed rather the want of discipline in earlier days than any aptitude for a more sustained and severe study'.[5] This perceptive judgement was borne out at numerous stages of Jenner's career. At all events Jenner returned to Berkeley, well aware of his tendency to indolence, as he confessed to a former schoolfriend: 'of all the habits... indolence is the most difficult to get rid of', and settled into the steady routine of life as a country doctor. In 1785 he bought the pleasant house near the church known as The Chantry, now a museum devoted to his life and work, and in 1788 married Catherine Kingscote. Their engagement had been prolonged for many years, perhaps because of the ill health from which she was seldom free. In the following year their first child, Edward, was born and seemed, as his father reported, 'remarkably healthy'.[6]

During this period Jenner had maintained contact with Hunter who found him useful as a source of specimens for his own research. Bats, hedgehogs, crows' nests, magpies' nests were all in demand for experiments that Hunter was conducting on the heat of animals' bodies in life and death. Letters passed back and forth, including at least one exchange on the subject of the cuckoo. 'I received yours,' Hunter wrote, 'as also the cuckoo's stomach. I should like a few more of them, for I find they do not all show the same thing'. These days, when the sound of a cuckoo is rare enough to bring the countryside to a halt while everyone listens, it is difficult to picture the time when Jenner's nephew Henry, his apprentice since 1783, could go on a five-mile ramble round the hedgerows of Berkeley every morning noting the locations and adaptation of the young cuckoos to their ruthlessly acquired foster homes. This information and his own observations enabled Jenner to put together a paper on the cuckoo that was sent to the Royal Society for publication in its *Transactions* but had to be hurriedly recalled. He had based his treatise on the assumption generally accepted at the time that the mother cuckoo ejected the rightful occupant from the nest she had commandeered. Jenner had belatedly established the far more astonishing fact that it is not the mother but the young cuckoo which, by means of an adaptation of its own body, turfs its foster parent's offspring out in order to make room for itself. A revised paper incorporating this discovery, which many ornithologists had difficulty in accepting, was included in the *Transactions* and in 1789 Jenner was made a Fellow of the Royal Society, an honour that, it has been suggested, probably carried less prestige in the eighteenth century than in later years. As Jenner learned to his discomfiture in due course, when the paper he submitted on cowpox as a preventive of smallpox was returned to him as being not up to standard, the members were not to be easily hoodwinked.

The antecedents of the paper are the subject of what Greenwood describes as a 'mythology', much of it traceable to Baron. According to his account it was in the mid-1770s, while Jenner was a teenager learning his trade as an apothecary in Sodbury, that his interest in cowpox was first aroused:

> [A] young woman came to seek advice; the subject of small-pox was mentioned in her presence: she immediately observed, 'I cannot take the disease, for I have had cow-pox.' This incident riveted the attention of Jenner. Young as he was […] he […] partly foresaw the vast consequences which were involved in so remarkable a phenomenon.

Later elaborations of the mythology have him brooding incessantly on the subject for the next thirty years until he first went into print with it in 1798. He seems on occasion to have consulted Hunter who is alleged on no very sound evidence to have referred to it in some of his public lectures. The medical men in Jenner's part of Gloucestershire also became very familiar with his preoccupation with the topic, and were, he admitted, not very enthusiastic.

'We have heard' (they would observe) 'of what you mention and have even seen examples which certainly do give some countenance to the notion to which you allude but we have all known cases of a perfectly different nature – many who were reported to have had the cow-pox having subsequently caught [...] the small-pox. The supposed prophylactic powers, probably, therefore, depend upon some peculiarity in the constitution of the individual who has escaped the small-pox and not on any efficacy of that disorder which they may have received from the cow. In short, the evidence is altogether so inconclusive and unsatisfactory that we can put no value on it, and cannot think that it will lead to anything but uncertainty and disappointment.'

Seldom can even the most polite scepticism have been expressed in so many words.

Jenner was not put off and continued to seek answers to the basic questions: why, and how, did cowpox prevent an attack of smallpox? By about 1780 he felt sufficiently sure that he was on the right track to confide in a close friend, Edward Gardner. During a long ride from Gloucester to Bristol he favoured Gardner with a full exposition of his train of thought and the almost overwhelming conclusion it seemed to point to, the possible extinction of smallpox world-wide. He concluded, Baron says, with words to the following effect:

Gardner, I have entrusted a most important matter to you, which I firmly believe will prove of essential benefit to the human race. I know you, and should not wish what I have stated to be brought into conversation: for should anything untoward turn up in my experiments I should be made, particularly by my medical brethren, the subject of ridicule, for I am the mark they all shoot at.[7]

A modern commentator finds it difficult to believe that the words were ever spoken and suggests that Baron 'even convinced Jenner in later years of events that never happened'; but there is no doubt that Gardner corroborated Baron's account of the conversation in evidence to a Parliamentary Committee of Inquiry, albeit more than twenty years later.

The puzzling word is 'experiments', for there is nothing to show what these might have been, or that Jenner did anything more practical than cogitate while pursuing his normal occupation as a country doctor. His principal activity seems to have been the collection of information from various sources of persons of all ages who had at some time allegedly contracted cowpox from the diseased udder of a cow and thereafter never suffered an attack of smallpox, but much of the evidence scarcely stood up to close examination. In some cases it consisted of little more than hearsay or uncertain memory, in others what was claimed to have been cowpox was more likely to have been mild smallpox, even a slight attack of which would, in the majority of cases, have conferred lifelong immunity from further attacks. The crucial test, if Jenner's grandiose theories were to become reality, would be to take matter from a pustule of a patient suffering from cowpox, inoculate with it the body of a person known for certain never to have had smallpox, and subsequently to attempt unsuccessfully to give them smallpox. The next step would be to ascertain whether the inoculated cowpox could be passed on to one or more further recipients, so as to set going a chain reaction from which ultimately, in theory, whole populations could be immunized and smallpox finally 'extirpated'.

Another sixteen years elapsed before Jenner could bring himself to attempt the necessary first step. In May 1796 Sarah Nelmes, the daughter of a farmer in the neighbourhood of Berkeley, showed what were indisputably the signs of cowpox on her hands after milking a cow suffering from the disease. Jenner took matter from one of the pustules with his lancet and transferred it to the arm of an eight-year-old boy called James Phipps, who in due course developed cowpox. Several weeks later he was inoculated with smallpox and failed to respond with even a modified form of the disease. This was the first successful example of what came to be called 'vaccination', a word coined by one of Jenner's friends from the Latin *vacca*, meaning a cow. To distinguish the two processes, inoculation for smallpox came to be known more frequently by the corresponding Latin-based term 'variolation'.

The success of this trial, in conjunction with the other material he had assembled, seemed to Jenner to provide sufficient support for his general conclusions, which he set out in the paper intended for publication in the *Philosophical Transactions*. He was much mortified when it was tactfully but firmly rejected on the ground that the evidence he had adduced was considered to be insufficiently conclusive to justify his claims for the prophylactic power of cowpox. After some tinkering with the manuscript, which did not materially improve it or meet the Royal Society's criticisms, Jenner published it himself in 1798 under the title *An Inquiry into the Cause and Effects of the VARIOLAE VACCINAE, a disease discovered in some of the Western Counties of England, particularly Gloucestershire, and known by the name of the Cow-pox.*

In the absence of the disease that its exploitation was intended to prevent, cowpox and the questions and disagreements it gave rise to are of interest today chiefly to epidemiologists, biologists, pathologists and other specialists. There is, we are assured by those who have investigated the subject, no way of knowing precisely what the disease was that Jenner studied, nor where it came from, or where, if anywhere, it lurks today. Much of the argument that followed the introduction of vaccination was based on false premises or few notions at all concerning why it behaved as it did: the elucidation of these mysteries had to wait until the early twentieth century.

On the other hand there were certain aspects of the cowpox controversy that reached far beyond the squabbles of the medical profession, ultimately affecting, sometimes seriously, the lives of every family in the country. The most significant of them arose directly from the doctrines set out in the comparatively small body of writings left behind by Jenner, a brief summary of which follows, beginning with the classic *Inquiry*.

The opening paragraphs of the work are worth recalling at some length because they incorporated a misunderstanding that had formed part of the foundation of Jenner's theory from the earliest days, and although he subsequently abandoned it, it was still being used to discredit him long after his death.

> The deviation of man from the state in which he was originally placed by nature seems to have proved to him a prolific source of disease. From the love of splendour, from the indulgence of luxury, and from his fondness for amusement, he has familiarised himself with a great number of animals which may not originally have been intended for his associates. There is a disease to which the horse, from his state of domestication, is frequently subject. The farriers have termed it the grease. It is an inflammation and swelling in the heel, from which issues matter possessing properties of a peculiar kind, which seems capable of generating a disease in the human body, which bears so strong a resemblance to the small-pox that I think it highly probable it may be the source of that disease.

This conviction had been growing in Jenner's mind for some years; perhaps not as far back as his long conversation with Gardner but, if Baron is to be believed, from 1787, when Jenner, while visiting a stable with his nephew, George, pointed to a horse's heels and said, 'There is the source of small-pox. I have much on that subject which I hope in due time to give to the world.'

The *Inquiry* continued with a description of the chain of events that, in Jenner's mind, linked the horse with what he later referred to as 'the speckled monster', i.e. smallpox:

> In this dairy country a great number of cows are kept, and the office of milking is performed indiscriminately by men and maid servants. One of the former having been appointed to apply dressings to the heels of a horse affected with the grease, and not paying due attention to cleanliness, incautiously bears his part in milking the cows, with some particles of the infectious matter adhering to his fingers. When this is the case it commonly happens that a disease is communicated to the cows and from the cows to the dairy maids. This disease has obtained the name of the cow-pox.

So far so good; but what is the route by which we travel from cowpox to smallpox?

> Morbid matter of various kinds, when absorbed into the system, may produce effects in some degree similar; but what renders the cowpox virus so extremely singular, is that the person who has been thus affected is for ever after secure from the infection of the small-pox; neither exposure to the variolous effluvia, nor the insertion of the matter under the skin [i.e. variolation] producing this distemper.

Jenner was, he had already informed a friend several years before the publication of the *Inquiry*, convinced of the truth of his assertion 'beyond the possibility of a denial'; but he was wrong. Denials in plenty, from colleagues and friends whom he couldn't argue against, convinced him after his treatise had appeared that grease was not the origin of smallpox. He never published a retraction or an apology for his error; he simply dropped all reference to the subject, and paid a stiff penalty posthumously when his reputation came under attack on numerous other counts. The only printed apology, tucked away in the Appendix to Volume Two of his biography, is shamefacedly offered by Baron:

> I take this opportunity of expressing my regret that I have employed the word grease in alluding to the disease in the horse. Variolae Equinae [smallpox of the horse] is the proper designation [...] It has no necessary connexion with the grease, though the

disorders frequently co-exist. This circumstance at first misled Dr Jenner, and it has caused much misapprehension and confusion.

Variolae Equinae is an indirect reference to the term *Variolae Vaccinae* which Jenner had coined and incorporated in the title of the *Inquiry* to express one of his fundamental beliefs. The implication is not that cows suffered from smallpox, which had always been recognized as a disease solely of human beings. What Jenner did believe, and clung to in the face of all opposition, was that smallpox and cowpox were, in Baron's phrase, 'modifications of the same distemper', and therefore, in employing vaccine lymph, 'we only make use of means to impregnate the constitution with the disease in its mildest instead of propagating it in its virulent and contagious form, as is done when small-pox is inoculated'. Elsewhere Baron set out what were claimed as the principal characteristics that distinguished 'small-pox of the cow':

> One of [its] properties is that it is an affection extremely mild in its nature and affords when it has regularly passed through its stages a complete immunity from subsequent attacks of small-pox as that disease itself does [...] But the property, of all others, which peculiarly distinguishes the Variolae Vaccinae from small-pox [...] is that they [*sic*] are not communicable by effluvia.

In brief, cowpox was safe, effective and not infectious; the vaccinated person was not, while passing through the disease, a danger to anyone else. Needless to say, this was an oversimplification of a complex problem and in a short essay, published in 1801, on *The Origin of the Vaccine Inoculation*, Jenner described some of the difficulties he had encountered in the course of his investigations. 'I found that some of those *who seemed to have undergone the cow pox*, nevertheless, on inoculation with the small-pox, felt its influence just the same as if no disease had been communicated to them by the cow.' This, as he put it, dampened but did not extinguish his ardour. Further inquiries showed that the cow was 'subject to some varieties of spontaneous eruptions on her teats', which produced sores on the hands of milkers who classed them all as 'the Cow Pox'. This led him to his famous distinction between '*true*' cowpox, the kind that worked, and '*spurious*' cowpox, all those that didn't. But no sooner was this obstacle removed than another took its place:

> There were not wanting instances to prove, that when the true cow pox broke out among the cattle at a dairy, a person who had

milked an infected animal, and had thereby apparently gone through the disease in common with others, was liable to receive the small pox afterwards.

This, by striking at the heart of his claim that cowpox was an infallible preventive of smallpox, 'gave a painful check to my fond and aspiring hopes'. But he reasoned that 'the operations of nature are generally uniform'; if one injection of cowpox matter behaved differently from others there must be a reason, and in due course he discovered what it was:

> The virus of cow pox was liable to undergo progressive changes from the same causes precisely as that of small pox: [...] when it was applied to the human skin in its degenerated state, it would produce the ulcerated effects in as great a degree as when it was not decomposed, and sometimes far greater; but having lost its *specific properties* it was incapable of producing that change upon the human frame which is required to render it unsusceptible of the variolous contagion...

The explanation may at first appear laboured but is in fact lucid and precise, and led to the formulation of Jenner's 'golden rule' governing the time at which lymph intended for vaccination should be taken from the cowpox pustule, which he insisted should be done at an early period of its formation. Although he has been criticized in later times for attempting to make the operation sound unnecessarily difficult, and for using disregard of the 'rule' as an all-purpose excuse for vaccinations that failed, it helps to explain why so much of what was ultimately passed off as vaccination proved to be useless.

* * *

There has been a certain amount of equivocation concerning Jenner's claims for cowpox inoculation. Baron, referring to the parliamentary debates that resulted in financial awards to Jenner, remarks,

> In these discussions we hear nothing of vaccination as an infallible preventive of small-pox. I am not sure whether the expression was ever used by Dr. Jenner himself. If he did use it he certainly very soon accompanied it with the necessary qualification. He may perhaps at the very outset have stated his opinion somewhat too decidedly, but no one can doubt that he, from the very beginning,

was possessed of the gauge by which he measured the virtue of vaccination. *'Duly and efficiently performed it will protect the constitution from subsequent attacks of small-pox as much as that disease itself will. I never expected that it would do more, and it will not, I believe do less.'*[8]

This passage is printed in italics in Baron's *Life*. Quoting it in his authoritative *Handbook of Vaccination* (1868), Edward Seaton adds his own comment:

Whatever phrase may be picked out of Jenner's writings here and there to show that he looked on the security which cow-pox would impart against small-pox as an *absolute*, that he believed the human system which had once felt genuine cow-pox was 'never afterwards, at any period of its existence assailable by small-pox', must be read with this limitation.[9]

Seaton was writing more than forty years after Jenner's death. Baron was Jenner's close friend and biographer. Of all the documents that passed through his hands he cannot have forgotten the *Proposals... for a Public Institution for Vaccine Inoculation*, based on the assurance that 'those who have gone through this mild disease are rendered perfectly safe from the contagion of the small-pox'.[10] No qualifications there; nor in the text of the 'humble petition of Edward Jenner [...] to the Honourable the Commons of the United Kingdom and Ireland in Parliament assembled', drawing attention to 'the great expense and anxiety he had suffered through his researches into vaccination', and praying for 'such remuneration as in their wisdom shall seem meet'. The service that he had performed for 'his countrymen and mankind in general' was the 'discovery of a disease [...] attended with the singular beneficial effect of rendering through life the person so inoculated perfectly secure from the infection of the small-pox'.[11] He could not have chosen a more formal and prominent occasion for so definitive a pronouncement and he could hardly complain if his adversaries, of whom he had plenty, should fasten on it, ignoring the limitation he later tried to draw round it.

For the rest of his life Jenner was plagued by reports and allegations, not all of them false or frivolous, of 'small-pox after cow-pox'. Disciples, sometimes over-enthusiastic, rallied to his defence. In 1804, for example, a surgeon practising in Portsmouth published the details of several cases of patients whom he had vaccinated and who had later returned to him suffering from smallpox; his concern in speaking publicly was to raise the issue of how long cowpox might be expected to stave off smallpox. One of Jenner's most fervent propagandists, James Ring, promptly replied with an immensely long tract under the defiant title: *An answer to Mr Goldson proving that vaccination is a permanent security against the small pox.*

Three years later, in a treatise with the promising title *A Popular View of Vaccine Inoculation*, Joseph Adams, physician to the Smallpox and Inoculation Hospitals, dealt with the subject in some depth. Taking for granted the analogy between smallpox and cowpox, and mentioning that the suspicion that cowpox was proving only a temporary security had first been raised in 1803, he asked in a chapter heading 'Is vaccination a security against the small pox?' and showed that at least at that time there was much to be said on both sides:

> Friends of vaccination urge with much truth that the small pox has occurred more than once in the same subject. Those on the other side who are candid enough to admit this assert that instances appear to be more numerous after the cow pox [...] the small pox has appeared after the cow pox in two different forms. In by far the most numerous instances so mild and deficient in many of its true characters, as to excite a doubt of the reality of the disease.
>
> In a very few instances [...] the small pox has occurred after vaccination in so serious a form as to threaten and even to be followed by fatal consequences. The question will then remain whether the same has not frequently happened after the small pox?

How, then, was the security of vaccination to be estimated, bearing in mind the uncertainty of the process?

> It must be confessed that the friends of vaccination have been much too forward in accounting for supposed failures by the imputation of an improper, or as they would often call it an ignorant, mode of conducting vaccination [...] it would be easy to show that the same objection may be started against variolous inoculation.

The controversy was not always conducted in so moderate a manner. In 1809 a surgeon in Scotland (dismissed by one critic as 'fretting in the obscurity of Musselburgh') published an *Inquiry into the anti-variolous power of vaccination*, in which he expressed the opinion, based on his own observations, that its virtue diminished as the distance from the period of vaccination increased: in three years its influence declined, and in five or six years hardly any security against smallpox remained. This view, allowing for some sharp differences over the number of years, was ultimately accepted by most authorities, and led to the practice of re-vaccination at the appropriate age, usually the onset of puberty. At the time of its publication the pamphlet and the correspondence it engendered, having been read by an authority it attacked, was 'tied up in red tape amongst the mass of papers which are allowed to rest'.

Incidents of this kind followed the recognized adversarial procedures of the medical and other professions, from which in due course something approximating to a generally acceptable truth will probably emerge, but some of the 'anti-vaccs', as Jenner called them, responded to the perceived threat to their own profitable activities with an uninhibited campaign of scurrilous lies and abuse. Among the recognized ringleaders, 'the renowned triumvirate' were Drs Squirrel, Rowley and Moseley, who, between them, cost Jenner much annoyance and anguish.

The essence of the argument of Squirrel, the pseudonym of John Jones, sometime apothecary at the Smallpox and Inoculation Hospitals, was summed up in the flamboyant title page of his pamphlet:

OBSERVATIONS addressed to the public in general on the COW-POX, showing that it originates in SCROFULA, commonly called the EVIL, illustrated with cases to prove that it is no security against the SMALL-POX. Also pointing out the dreadful consequences of this new disease, so recently, and rashly, introduced into the human constitution. To which are added observations on the SMALL-POX INOCULATION, proving it to be more beneficial to society than the vaccine.

The 'evil' was tuberculosis, the 'King's Evil', so called because of the belief that being touched by the King was a cure for it. Among other shafts that he directed against Jenner and the leaders of the medical profession, Squirrel argued that inoculation had never been the province of physicians. They considered it much beneath them, and even thought themselves degraded in performing the operation; nor was it deemed necessary that they should attend to the progress of the disease; and though in other respects they might be extremely well acquainted with the profession of medicine in general, yet with regard to inoculation in particular 'they had not practice sufficient to furnish them with an adequate knowledge of the subject'. They were not in his view qualified to make any innovation in a profession which had always been practised by apothecaries and surgeons, 'the only men in this country possessing any claims to a real judgment'.

For the effect of cowpox on the 'human condition' we may turn to William Rowley, a member of the Royal College of Physicians and various other institutions, the title page of whose treatise, though typographically less eye-catching than Squirrel's, is more informative:

> *Cow-Pox Inoculation no security against Small-Pox Infection. With above 500 proofs of failure* [...] *To which are added the modes of treating the Beastly new diseases produced from Cow Pox* [sic]... [with] *500 dreadful cases of small-pox after vaccination: or* [i.e. showing that vaccination didn't work]

Cow-Pox Mange	Cow-Pox Evil or abscess
Cow-Pox Ulcers	Cow-Pox mortification etc.

> *with the author's certain, experienced and successful mode of Inoculating for the Small-Pox, which now becomes necessary from Cow-Pox failures etc.*

A journeyman apothecary is said to have confessed that he was one of a number of persons paid by Rowley for finding out 'cases', and that when other sources failed he 'forged names, addresses and disasters, at his own hazard for Rowley's love of miseries rendered him the dupe of his informer'.

'The Small-Pox,' Rowley asserted,

> is a visitation from God, and originated in man, but the Cow Pox is produced by presumptuous, impious man: the former heaven ordained, the latter is, perhaps, a daring and profane violation of our holy religion. Heaven seems daily to justify this supposition from the dreadful calamities Cow Pox has occasioned.

It seems to have been Rowley who introduced to the world the Ox-Faced Boy, who became a symbol of the horrors to be apprehended from vaccination. 'Dr Moseley [...] saw the case of the ox-faced boy by my desire. He observed to me, that the boy's face seemed to be in a state of transforming and assuming the visage of a cow' (gender seems to have given Rowley a certain amount of trouble). An etching of the unfortunate youth who, if he existed, may have been suffering from some totally unrelated disease was the inspiration for cartoons by Gillray and others depicting victims in the process of being what Peter Quince would have called 'translated'.

Benjamin Moseley was one of the earliest opponents of vaccination, having fired off the first shots in January 1799, less than a year after the publication of Jenner's *Inquiry*. Physician to the Royal Military College in Chelsea and member of various professional institutions, he had spent some years in the West Indies and boasted that there, and in Europe, he had 'inoculated several thousands [and] never lost a patient'. A resident of Jamaica remained unimpressed by the 'pompous' Dr Moseley: '[he] practised at Kingston in this island, and it is a well-known fact that his practice was extremely limited, and that he was much more devoted to music than medicine.'

Judging by his prose style Moseley was indeed given to pomposity, but by steering clear of the hysteria and wild invective of the average 'anti-vacc' he succeeded in being more effective in his criticism. He was the author of many dissertations, on tropical diseases, on sugar, on coffee, on tea; but his main contribution to the vaccination controversy was *A Treatise on the Lues Bovilla, or Cow Pox*. Taking its epigraph from the New Testament – 'Father, forgive them for they know not what they do' – it combined the usual defence of inoculation and assault on vaccination with a good deal of heavy-handed ridicule at the expense of the pro-vaccination school. His main themes were bestiality and the rights of parents, both of them long runners in the latter part of the century:

Accidents in the inoculated small-pox are uncommon; and we all know from experience that [that] disease, properly treated, leaves nothing after it injurious to the constitution.

Can anyone say what may be the consequences of introducing a *bestial* humour into the human frame, after a long lapse of years? Who knows, besides, what ideas may rise, in the course of time, from a *brutal* fever having excited its incongruous impressions on the brain? Who knows, also, but that the human character may undergo strange mutations from *quadrupedan* sympathy; and that some modern Pasiphaë may rival the fables of old.

'This,' he conceded, was 'serious trifling', but there was no trifling when it came to the part played by doctors, who set the example 'with a spirit worthy of the Agricultural Society, by experimenting with their own flock':

The doctors renounced all discussion, concerning the rights of parents, to take what liberty they pleased with their infants, whose sympathies and antipathies, as they cannot be known, they determined to be proper objects for experiment.

It was never agitated to what extent of conscience a parent might go when children cannot judge for themselves: know nothing of the game that is playing, and are compelled into a lottery, where there can be no losers but themselves.

Parents were not told that their children, more advanced in years, would be submitted to the continual dread of the smallpox

and that they might not be able to get rid of this dread, by small-pox inoculation, as formerly, or by going into infected company – their state of susceptibility being suspended by the cow-pox poison, while its uncertain action remained in their constitutions.

There was no suspicion excited at the time, in the minds of parents, that before six years should elapse, doubting of the security of the cow-pox, their alarms would induce them to expose their children to new vexation, to undo what they had done.

The antics of the more unscrupulous anti-vaccs caused Jenner much anxiety and agitation, most of it unnecessary since the lower classes were unlikely to come across their diatribes and in any case, if they took any precaution at all against smallpox, for themselves or their children, they were more likely to choose variolation, which they were familiar with, in preference to vaccination which for various reasons they didn't like the sound of or trust. The great majority of Jenner's professional colleagues took his side in the argument with an alacrity that at this distance appears almost incomprehensible. In July 1800, after barely two years in which to undertake anything like a searching test of Jenner's claims, an impressive roll-call of 70 or so of the leading lights put their names to an uncompromising 'testimonial in favour of the cow-pox':

Many unfounded reports having been circulated which have a tendency to prejudice the public against inoculation of the cow-pox: we the undersigned physicians and surgeons think it our duty to declare our opinion that those persons who have had the cow-pox are perfectly secure from the future infection of the small-pox.

We also declare that the inoculated cow-pox is a much milder and safer disease than the inoculated small-pox.[12]

A strange omission in the circumstances is any reference to one of the least controversial and most beneficial characteristics of cowpox, that unlike smallpox it was not contagious. One reason for the almost indecent haste with which the more responsible members of the profession rushed into their declaration may have been an urgent desire to dissociate themselves from the discredited smallpox inoculation. It was noticed and commented upon that some of the most enthusiastic vaccinators had not long previously been among the most ardent variolators, and were now advocates of legislation to prohibit the smallpox inoculation they had so recently been practising. The alarm that this development created is apparent in a passage from Moseley's pamphlet:

> It surpasses all rational belief that some enthusiasts were so transported from their sober senses as to meditate an application for the interference of Parliament to prevent all further inoculation for the small-pox under the severest pains and penalties. Others, not stopping here, and before they could possibly know whether cowpox would prove a blessing or a curse, wanted this experiment in medicine to make a part in parental duty, and to be blended in the House of God with our duties to the Supreme Being. The Archbishop of Canterbury was even applied to, petitioning his Grace to recommend the cow-pox to the bishops; desiring at the same time that they would enjoin the clergy in their respective dioceses to preach the divine attributes from their pulpits.

The clergy responded not merely by preaching cowpox inoculation but by practising it, as with the introduction of smallpox inoculation eighty years earlier. A parson in Lancashire was reported to have carried out more than 3,000 vaccinations. Another, in whose parish there was no medical practitioner, inoculated 'upwards of 300'. The rector of a parish in Surrey who was also a magistrate 'had not thought it any disparagement of his rank, to inoculate his poor neighbours with his own hands'. Nor were fashionable ladies backward in taking on their share of the burden. A lady of Portman Square in London, with another lady, inoculated 1,300 persons in the north of England. Miss Bayley of Hope near Manchester had notched up a total of 2,600 vaccinations by 1805. Dr Willan, author of a *Treatise on Vaccination*, estimated that 10,000 or perhaps 12,000 'private individuals taking up the lancet, [had] extended the benefits [...] of vaccination to every corner of the land'. William Cobbett, a predictable opponent of vaccination, chiefly on account of its 'beastliness' commented drily on the situation in the south of England where,

the quackery having been sanctioned by King, Lords and

Commons spread over the country like a pestilence borne by the winds. 'Gentlemen and Ladies' made the commodity a pocket companion, and if a cottager's child (in Hampshire at least) ever seen by them on a common, were not pretty quick in taking to its heels, it had to carry off more or less of the disease of the cow. One would have thought that one-half of the cows in England must have been tapped to get at such a quantity of the stuff.[13]

The sad truth was that most of this enthusiasm was wasted because, with the exception of a limited number of amateurs whom Jenner personally instructed, the 'golden rule', which was the foundation of good vaccinating technique, was either unknown or ignored: 'Never take matter [from a donor] after the eighth or ninth day of the disease, or after the areola round the pustule has fully formed'. Failure to observe this strict injunction was responsible for much of the derided 'spurious cowpox' that he warned against. He deplored the state of affairs in a letter to Moore:

Vaccination at its commencement fell into the hands of many who knew little more about it than its mere outline. One grave error, which was almost universal at the time was making one puncture only, and consequently only one vesicle [...] and from this (the only source of security to the constitution) as much fluid was taken day after day as it would afford: nevertheless it was unreasonably expected that no mischief would ensue [...] I have taken a world of pains to correct this abuse, but still, to my knowledge, it is going on and particularly among the faculty in town.[14]

This may be a coded reference to one of a series of altercations in which he became embroiled and which cast shadows over his later years. The details lie outside the scope of the present work but the main events can be summarized.

In November 1798 Jenner received a letter praising the *Inquiry* to the skies and concluding, 'Your name will live on in the memory of mankind as long as men possess gratitude for service and respect for benefactors; and if I can but get *matter* [i.e. vaccine lymph] I am much mistaken if I do not make you live for ever.'[15] The writer was Dr George Pearson, physician to St George's Hospital in London. Jenner must have been much gratified by this response to the *Inquiry*, but when he should have been capitalizing on it with further research into the subject he surrendered instead to that indolence he had accused himself of in days gone by, allowing smarter operators to get ahead of him with the work he had left undone. Early in 1799 he began to hear what the man who was going to 'make him live for ever' had been up to. Pearson had sent questionnaires to practitioners countrywide asking for their opinions and experience of cowpox. In March Jenner's nephew, George, wrote to him, 'Dr Pearson is going to send circular letters to the medical gentlemen to let them know that he will supply them with cow-pox matter upon their application to him, by which means he will be the chief person known in the business and consequently deprive you of that merit, or at least a great deal of it which is so justly your due'.[16] Jenner's proposed response in a letter to his old friend Gardner was 'should not some neatly-drawn paragraphs appear from time to time in the public prints, by no means reflecting on the conduct of P. but just to keep the idea publicly alive that P. was not the author of the discovery – I mean cow-pox inoculation'.[17]

Meanwhile Woodville, physician to the Smallpox and Inoculation hospitals, had been carrying out trials with cowpox matter collected from dairy farms in the neighbourhood of London. These had resulted in the appearance of what were fairly obviously smallpox pustules on the bodies of the chosen patients, from which the experimenter concluded, and said publicly, that cowpox did not, to say the least, possess all the characteristics that Jenner claimed for it. Jenner in some perturbation tactfully suggested that to carry out trials of cowpox on premises where smallpox patients were being treated, and others inoculated, was a procedure calculated to risk contaminating the cowpox samples with smallpox. Woodville huffily conceded that there might be some force in the argument but in the meantime, owing to a recurrent shortage of cowpox matter, some of his samples had found their way into surgeries across the country, where they were used for inoculations that, by the arm-to-arm process, were used for further inoculations. This gave rise to a theory that held sway in some quarters until modern times that all subsequent immunity allegedly due to vaccination with cowpox matter had in fact been due to inoculation with smallpox matter. The charge has been examined at some length by Baxby, who finds no substance in it.[18]

Towards the end of 1799 Jenner received notification from Pearson of the progress being made 'in the institution of a charity for inoculating the vaccine pock' free of charge to the poor. The promoters had got 'very high patronage', including members of the royal family, and it had occurred to Pearson that it might not be disagreeable to Jenner to become 'an extra corresponding physician', at no expense beyond a guinea a year as a subscriber. His presence would not be required in town. Jenner's response was predictable. He found it 'somewhat extraordinary' that an institution formed for the purpose of inoculating the cowpox should have been set on foot without his receiving 'the most distant intimation of it'. He begged leave 'to decline the *honour* intended me', and took no further part in the institution's proceedings. Dixon believes that Pearson and Woodville had a certain amount of right on their side, because Jenner had shown himself 'an impossible man to work with'; at the same time he attributes to Jenner 'ethical standards far ahead of his time', which begs the question, by what criteria should the ethical standards of Pearson and Woodville be judged?

After much negotiation, which drew Jenner to London for a while, the high patronage was withdrawn from Pearson's (and Woodville's) Cowpock Institution and transferred to a Royal Jennerian Society, whose object was 'to see the practice of vaccination fixed on a firm basis': the King was its patron and Jenner its president.

In spite of Jenner's protestation that he was not short of money and only wanted a quiet life, there was a feeling among his supporters that his work for the promotion of vaccination had not been adequately acknowledged and that he was bound to be out of pocket because he had financed it largely from his own resources. The outcome was the petition to Parliament, referred to above, that he was persuaded to draw up. A committee of members was appointed in March 1802 to assess the claims made on behalf of vaccination and Jenner's alleged contribution to its development.[19]

The committee, chaired by Admiral Berkeley, one of Jenner's unofficial patrons, broke with precedent where petitions were concerned by hearing testimony from hostile witnesses, notably Pearson, to the effect that they had in some way anticipated Jenner's research, and even practised inoculation with cowpox before he did, although they had not studied the subject systematically. The committee rejected these allegations and accepted the view epitomized in the words of a medical witness that Jenner's work on cowpox inoculation represented 'the greatest discovery ever made in the practice of physic for the preservation of human life', and that Jenner could have made at least £10,000 a year by keeping the secret of successful vaccination to himself. The precedent of Sutton was frequently quoted, although Sutton had amassed his fortune in spite of his methods becoming common knowledge.

The report of the investigating committee went forward to a committee of the whole House of Commons where its recommendations were debated on 2 June. Admiral Berkeley proposed and defended a grant to Jenner of £10,000, which was approved by speaker after speaker, with the exception of a small minority who thought the sum was inadequate. The Chancellor of the Exchequer, while agreeing that cowpox inoculation was 'one of the most important discoveries to human society that was made since the creation of man', did not think himself justified under the circumstances in accepting an amendment that would have increased the proposed grant to £20,000. When the House divided on a motion that 'the words £10,000 do stand part of the resolution' the Ayes had it by 59 votes to the Noes 56. It was pointed out that, allowing for about £6,000 of his own money that Jenner had already spent, plus the cost of the petition, he was little better off. Four years later Parliament voted him a further £20,000.

By that time it was becoming apparent that all was not well with the Royal Jennerian Society. Among the staff appointed at its inception was Dr John Walker as resident inoculator and medical secretary. As time went by Dr Walker's working methods began to infringe the basic Jennerian principles so flagrantly that Jenner finally insisted on his dismissal. Typical of his alleged procedures was his vaccination, in both arms, of Laura Watkins,

> daughter of a gentleman of distinguished character in the literary world. On the eighth day, when the areola was as large as a shilling, and when he ought not to have taken matter at all, unless in a case of absolute necessity, Dr Walker pricked the vesicle on the right arm in several places, totally removed the cuticle from its surface and wiped out the sore with the skirt of the child's frock. He then charged two lancets, three or four vaccinators, and a considerable number of glasses [flat plates for the preservation of lymph in dried form]. When charging the glasses he first drew the flat surface of them over the sore and then scraped up most of the matter with their edges.[20]

After a good deal of vicious and much publicized in-fighting Walker resigned and set up in opposition the London Vaccine Institution, which prospered while the Jennerian Society steadily declined and finally expired in 1809.

A problem with vaccination was the tendency of cowpox to disappear from the countryside from time to time for no known reason, reappearing just as inexplicably in due course. To overcome the difficulty the government created a National Vaccine Board consisting of the senior officials of the Royal Colleges of Physicians and Surgeons, which in turn set up a National Vaccine Establishment whose function was to collect surplus vaccine matter from public vaccination stations opened in large towns and cities to supersede the charitable institutions, and despatch it free in dried form to applicants who would reconstitute it for use in their own surgeries. Dried lymph was generally regarded as inferior to the moist variety obtained directly from the donor's arm, but was clearly better than nothing. Sir Lucas Pepys, president of the Royal College of Physicians, who was said to have been 'no friend to vaccination' but whose grandson Jenner had vaccinated, offered Jenner the post of director of the establishment. Jenner accepted and submitted a list of those whom he would like to appoint to his staff. When it was returned to him with all but one of his nominees deleted he resigned, and the post went to James Moore, frequently quoted above, a member of the College, surgeon of the second regiment of Life Guards and brother of the more illustrious Sir John Moore, the story of whose clandestine nocturnal obsequies following the battle of Corunna is the subject of a once famous poem.

In 1813 Oxford University conferred on Jenner the honorary degree of MD by diploma, which left only one significant professional distinction that had not come his way. Although he had obtained his MD from St Andrews, which qualified him to practise in most places throughout the country, he had never gained membership of the Royal College of Physicians, without which he was not permitted to practise in London and its immediate environs. In 1814 he applied for membership and was reminded that this could only be granted to candidates who passed the College's written examination, which included papers in Latin and Greek. Jenner was now in his mid-sixties with a worldwide reputation, the recipient of honours from countless learned institutions, and felt that some dispensation might be granted in his favour. The College replied that rules were rules. 'In my youth,' Jenner wrote to a friend,

> I went through the ordinary course of a classical education, obtained a tolerable proficiency in the Latin language, and got a smattering of Greek, but the greater part of it has long since transmigrated into heads better suited for its cultivation. At my time of life to set about brushing up would be irksome to me beyond measure [...] I would not do it for a diadem [...] I would not do it for John Hunter's museum, and that you will allow is no trifle.[21]

His disgust and contempt for the upper echelons of his profession were palpable and following the death of his invalid wife in the following year he rarely left Berkeley for the rest of his life.

The product of a modest rural background, Jenner had always been temperamentally ill-equipped for the cut and thrust of what was, in his day, a disorganized and ruthlessly competitive profession. He now withdrew into the 'cottage-ish' existence he had always preferred, keeping up a vast correspondence as 'vaccine clerk to the world' and finding release in an otherwise melancholy old age by immersing himself in his civic duties as mayor and magistrate of 'our good town of Berkeley'.

'I found him one day,' Baron recalled,

> sitting with a brother justice in a narrow, dark, tobacco-flavoured room, listening to parish business of all sorts. The door was surrounded by a scolding, brawling mob. A fat overseer of the poor was endeavouring to moderate their noise, but they neither heeded his authority nor that of their worships [...] He said to me, 'is this not too bad? I am the only acting magistrate in this place and I am really harassed to death...'[22]

However, Jenner was not so completely harassed as to prevent him from finding time to vaccinate his neighbours and their children at regular sessions in the rustic structure he called the Temple of Vaccinia, which was built for him and still survives in the garden of the Chantry.

Jenner died in 1823. The last words he wrote, as far as Baron could discover, were scribbled on the back of a letter and perhaps intended for a reply to the correspondent:

> My opinion of vaccination is precisely as it was when I first promulgated the discovery. It is not in the least strengthened by any event that has happened, for it could gain no strength; it is not in the least weakened, for if the failures you speak of had not happened, the truth of my assertions respecting those coincidences which occasioned them would not have been made out.[23]

CHAPTER 7

THE SPECKLED MONSTER

After the great surge of smallpox during the last quarter of the eighteenth century the disease relaxed its grip somewhat in the earlier years of the nineteenth, and the efforts of the medical profession were directed largely to weaning the lower classes away from variolation and selling them vaccination. The task was not easy; as Baron commented, the adoption by so many reputable medical men of vaccination left the field clear for the more unscrupulous practitioners who 'took up the small-pox lancet and disseminated the disease in a very frightful manner'.

The profession did its best to fight back. In 1805 the Medical Council of the Royal Jennerian Society appointed a committee of 25 members to investigate cases that had excited prejudices against vaccination and also the 'evidence respecting instances of small-pox alleged to have occurred twice in the same person'. The committee found that most of the alleged failures were 'either wholly unfounded or greatly misrepresented'; that 'nothwithstanding the most incontestable proofs of such misrepresentations, a few medical men have persisted in repeatedly bringing the same unfounded reports [...] before the public; then perversely and disingenuously labouring to excite prejudices against vaccination'; that 'many persons have been declared duly vaccinated, when the operation was performed in a very negligent and unskilful manner'; that 'the Medical Council are fully convinced that the failure of vaccination as a preventive of the small-pox, is a *very rare* occurrence'; that 'a few instances of failure either in the inoculation of the cow-pox as of the small-pox, ought not to be considered as objections to either practice, but merely as deviations from the usual course of nature'; that 'it appears to the Medical Council that the cow-pox is generally mild and harmless in its effects';[1] with much more in the same vein, concluding with a *solemn Declaration*, signed by 50 members of the Medical Council:

That, in their opinion [...] mankind have already derived great and incalculable benefit from the discovery of vaccination: and it is their full belief that the sanguine expectations of advantage, and security, which have been formed from the inoculation of the cow-pox, will be ultimately and completely fulfilled.[2]

This conclusion, promulgated by confessed adherents to the cause of Jenner and vaccination, could be dismissed as simply an expression of prejudice, but less than a year later the same issues were raised in the House of Commons. Lord Henry Petty, the Chancellor of the Exchequer, moved that

an address to His Majesty should be voted by the House, praying that his Royal College of Physicians be requested to inquire into the progress of vaccine inoculation, and to assign the causes of its success having been retarded throughout the United Kingdom, in order that their report may be made to this House of Parliament and that we may take the most proper means of publishing it to the inhabitants at large.[3]

The proposal was agreed to and the College set itself to go over much the same ground, but with an ardour and conviction in support of vaccination that made the Jennerian Society appear almost timid by comparison. Vaccination appeared to be in general perfectly safe. The security it offered against the smallpox, 'if not absolutely perfect, is as nearly so as can be expected from any human discovery [...] it appears that there are not nearly so many failures in a given number of vaccinated persons as there are deaths in an equal number of persons inoculated for the smallpox'. On the basis of its investigations it felt itself authorized to state 'that a body of evidence so large, so temperate and so consistent, was perhaps never before collected upon any medical question'. In a passage that it subsequently had reason to regret the College's report affirmed categorically that 'the opinion that vaccination affords but a temporary security is supported by no analogy in nature nor by the facts which have hitherto occurred'. In view of all the circumstances the College felt that it was its duty 'strongly to recommend the practice of vaccination'. It recognized, however, the nature of the difficulties that operated against the successful introduction of vaccination among those who were most in need of it:

The lower orders of society can hardly be induced to adopt precautions against evils which may be at a distance; nor can it be expected from them, if these precautions are attended with expense. Unless, therefore, from the immediate dread of epidemic small-pox, neither vaccination nor inoculation appear at any time to have been general, and when the cause of terror has passed by, the public have again relapsed into a state of indifference and apathy, and the salutary practice has come to a stand.[4]

A long-term cure for this 'evil in human nature' was not easy to find, but the report had two interim suggestions to offer: 'Were encouragement given to vaccination by offering it free of charge to the poorer classes, there is little doubt but it would in time supersede the inoculation for the small-pox, and thereby various sources of the variolous infection would be cut off.' This revolutionary proposal had to wait more than thirty years before government could be persuaded to act on it. In the meantime there was the problem of those who, for whatever reason, 'preferred the (inoculated) small-pox to the vaccine disease', thereby ensuring 'the constant recurrence of the natural small-pox'. The solution to the problem had been obvious to Jenner from the beginning:

> The small-pox rages at this time in the metropolis with desolating fury. We have the means in our power of stopping the calamity. Why not use them? [...] We bar the door against foreign plagues by our laws of quarantine, whilst the greatest domestic plague that ever infested us is suffered to advance without controul. Would it not be possible for the Legislature to interfere in the cause of suffering humanity?[5]

The suggestion was taken up in appropriately deferential terms by the report of the College of Physicians: might it not be proper for the Legislature, 'to adopt, in its wisdom, some measure by which those who still, from terror or prejudice, prefer the small-pox to the vaccine disease [...] may be prevented from doing mischief to their neighbours?'

Emboldened, presumably, by the College's endorsement of vaccination and perhaps by the further grant of £20,000 that the Commons had agreed to award him in recompense for his great and successful exertions, Jenner asked for an interview with the Prime Minister, Spencer Percival, with results that he gloomily communicated to Lettsom:

> I solicited this honour with the sole view of inquiring whether it was the intention of government to give a check to the licentious

manner in which small-pox inoculation is at the present time conducted in the metropolis. I instanced the mortality it occasioned in language as forcible as I could utter, and showed him clearly that it was the great source from which this pest was disseminated through the country as well as through the town. But, alas! all I said availed nothing; and the speckled monster is still to have the liberty that the Small-pox hospital, the delusions of Moseley, and the caprices and prejudices of the misguided poor, can possibly give him. I cannot express to you the chagrin and disappointment I felt at this interview.[6]

In 1810 the *Edinburgh Review* devoted two articles to a survey of a clutch of pamphlets on the general topic of vaccination, concluding with a summary of the arguments for and against the use of compulsion as a weapon in the fight to 'exterminate' the disease. Identifying public apathy or indifference as the most powerful obstacle to the progress of vaccination, the *Review* faced the crucial question, how could this apathy be overcome?

Are we [...] to use any other means than mere advice and example? Are we to have recourse to legislative measures? These are grave political questions in regard to which the present and late rulers of the state have expressed different opinions; Mr Percival conceiving that more evil than good would result from any measure of coercion; and Lord H. Petty taking a very different, and, we are inclined to think, a more correct view of the subject. 'Although compulsion be odious, and while it calls on mankind to be active against their will, yet while it goes no farther than to forbid that which is hurtful to others, I think that a state has not only a right but a duty to enforce it.'[7]

Thirty years later the opponents of smallpox inoculation won their case, but compulsory vaccination was even then scarcely considered. Peel, when Prime Minister, was reputed to have said that vaccination, if made compulsory, 'would be so opposite to the mental habits of the British people and to the freedom of opinion in which they glorified' that he could be no party to such compulsion.[8]

While the legislature and the intellectual elite were debating these grave political and philosophical issues it was left largely to the rank and file of the medical profession to bring to the attention of the lower classes, who on the whole did not read *Hansard*, the benefits they were missing by not espousing vaccination. One result was a spate of handbills and posters typified by a widely circulated *Address to the Poor* issued by the members of a charitable dispensary in Manchester:

> THE experience of several years has fully proved that inoculation for the COW-POX is a *certain preservative against* the SMALL-POX and is so safe and mild a disorder, when compared with the inoculated small-pox, that it has been generally introduced among the better-informed, and more wealthy inhabitants, both of the Kingdom and of various parts of Europe. In order therefore to impress strongly on the minds of the poor the usefulness and superior advantage of this new plan of inoculation the medical gentlemen whose signatures are annexed belonging to these charities have thought it their duty to state in this public manner the following observations for the serious perusal of all those poor persons who feel a proper affection for their offspring and who are desirous of promoting their own interest and comfort.[9]

Here followed a list of eleven advantages of vaccination over variolation:

> The prejudices of the poor against inoculation for the small-pox have often been lamented, but if they suffer unjust prejudices to prevent their laying hold of the advantages now offered to them by the inoculation of the cow-pox, they will neglect the performance of a duty they owe to themselves, to their families and to society at large. – For surely it is little less than criminal to expose their helpless children to the attack of so terrible and fatal a malady as the SMALL-POX when it may be readily avoided by the inoculation of so mild, simple and safe a disease as that of the COW-POX.

One cannot help feeling that the medical gentlemen of Manchester could have learned a trick or two from the Reverend Robert Houlton when it came to the art of inducing parental guilt and the knack of catching and holding the attention of the poor.

Smallpox and cowpox may have been, as Jenner maintained, different aspects of the same distemper, but from the point of view not only of the poor but of squeamish persons from all classes of society, there appeared to be one fundamental difference between them. Smallpox was a human disease, familiar to everyone. The poor in particular had learned by long experience to live with it, and by the early nineteenth century, through the Suttonian system that had filtered down to them, had become acquainted with a cheap and fairly reliable way of staving off its worst effects. Cowpox, however you looked at it, was a disease of animals, in the most literal sense 'bestial'; according to a speaker in the House of Lords in 1814, even the 'higher orders' had for some time been 'reluctant to introduce vaccination into their families' and might conclude that it would appear a 'harsh and arbitrary measure to lay the poor under the necessity of adopting the practice'. Moreover, you couldn't be sure what other 'bestial humours' the medical gentlemen might be injecting into your child's body along with the 'vaccine matter'. Farm workers knew about the disease that broke out on a cow's teats and thought little of it; it came, gave them little trouble, and went, leaving them, they hoped, immune to smallpox. For the city dwellers who, even when the countryside round London began at Gray's Inn Road or Highgate, had probably never seen milk being taken from a cow, the notion that the animal from which it was derived could be tainted with some nasty disease might be abhorrent even amid the normal squalor of their daily lives. The association of 'cow' with 'pox' was a turn-off, which promoters of vaccination did their best to counteract – not always with terminology calculated to get through to the ordinary citizen. Thus, Lettsom:

> An animal whose lactiferous fountains afford in our infancy a substitute for those of the parent, and from which we draw a considerable portion of our nutriment, is destined by the sagacity of one enlightened philosopher to protect the human species from the most loathsome and noxious disease to which it is subjected.[10]

John Ring, one of Jenner's most ardent disciples, was even more emphatic:

> Who could have imagined that a prejudice would arise in any human mind against the vaccine virus, on account of its being a bestial humour? That omnigenous mass, the human body, is formed by the conflux of all sorts of humours, from all sorts of animals, as well as vegetables, and not likely to be tainted by the juices of an animal whose food is the herb of the field, whose beverage is the limpid stream [...] The nature of matter cannot be bad when its effects are good; and to reject a benefit on account of its bestial origin is to betray a want of reason, more than bestial. The brute creation, in the choice of good and evil, are guided by an instinct that may put our boasted human reason to the blush![11]

James Moore, in *A Reply to the Anti-Vaccinists*, carried this line of argument to what must have seemed to many readers a horrifying and unacceptable conclusion:

The first objection which was urged against vaccination still continues a favourite one, namely that it is shocking even to the imagination to contaminate human beings with a bestial distemper. It requires, however, but little reflection to perceive that this is merely an imaginary objection. Few people are ignorant of this melancholy fact, that the most diseased animal in nature is man. Who would not think it a happy exchange, to barter the dreadful diseases we are infested with, for the milder indisposition incident to cows? Consider, for an instant, a few species of the numerous classes of human maladies. What surgeon, without horror, can recall to his memory the destructive progress and miserable termination of scrophula and cancer? or who, without disgust, can recollect the loathsome ulcers which break out in that infectious disease which poisons the breath, deforms the countenance, and corrodes the bones?[12]

Following the enumeration of the symptoms of syphilis and the vivid evocation of a typical case of confluent smallpox, Moore concludes: 'It is surely not in point of health that we can boast of a superiority over other animals'.

However sincerely and passionately the defenders of vaccination expressed themselves they made little impression at the time on their intended audience, who were unlikely to have read them anyway; and they would surely have greeted with bewilderment the savage rhetoric with which the disease of the cow and its promoters were still being denounced half a century after their deaths.

Particularly galling for Jenner as the years passed by was his unenviable role as a prophet without honour in his own country. European states banned inoculation with smallpox, beginning with Russia in 1805. Vaccination was made compulsory in Bavaria in 1807, Denmark in 1810 and Russia in 1812. Baron quotes at length the regulations issued in 1818 by the King of Wirtemburgh [*sic*] following several years of severe smallpox epidemics:

Every child must be vaccinated before it has completed its third year, under a penalty *annually* levied on its parents as long as the omission continues; and if the operation fail it must be repeated every three months until a third trial. No person to be received into any school, college or charitable institution; be bound apprentice to any trade; or hold any public office, who has not been vaccinated. When small-pox appears all those liable to take it must be vaccinated without delay [...] The superintendence of vaccination is limited to medical men [...] and a fine is levied on all who undertake to vaccinate without being duly qualified...[13]

Variolous inoculation was prohibited when smallpox was not present, and when it was, 'the practice can only be done by a medical man and under conditions of seclusion to prevent the disease from spreading'.

In Britain at this date inpatients in smallpox hospitals and charitable institutions were still being inoculated for smallpox: a bill brought forward in 1807 to forbid the practice made no progress and another in 1813, though not so stringent, was in the end no more successful. Promoted by the National Vaccine Board in response to an alarming rise in cases of smallpox in London, it was introduced in the House of Lords by Lord Boringdon. Its purpose was to regulate rather than ban smallpox inoculation and to ensure that if parents chose the older method in preference to vaccination the surrounding neighbourhood should, as far as possible, be protected from the spread of contagion. Among the opponents of the bill, without whose support it stood little chance of acceptance, were the Lord Chancellor, Lord Eldon, and the Lord Chief Justice, Lord Ellenborough, who held that the common law provided all the necessary safeguards. Ellenborough also let it be known, to Jenner's dismay, that he remained unconvinced that vaccination offered lifelong protection from smallpox. In these circumstances the bill, which even Baron conceded was 'rather a crude measure', was dropped. A new bill, which would have made vaccination compulsory for the poor, met a similar fate in 1814.

Within a few years the speckled monster, which had in general lain dormant since the turn of the century, roused itself and went on the offensive, stimulating a corresponding revival of variolation. Among the localities affected was the city of Norwich where smallpox, which had been endemic to a certain degree among the poor, erupted in 1819 into an epidemic that, in the words of a local parson, John Crosse, caused 'the most extreme destruction of human life that has ever, I believe, taken place in Norwich in the same space of time from any other cause than the plague'. Crosse estimated that considerably above 3,000 persons, or about one-thirteenth of the population of the city, had smallpox in the course of the year. Of the 530 deaths recorded, 260 were two years of age or under, 132 in the age group from two to four, and 86 from four years to six.

Crosse claimed that vaccination, introduced into Norwich soon after its discovery, was adopted by all the better classes of society and by 1806 had become so general that variolous inoculation was almost entirely 'discontinued, discountenanced and avoided by every respectable medical man'. The situation less than twenty years on was vastly different. Crosse himself attended 200 cases of smallpox and was able to observe how little headway had been made among the poor since Sydenham's day:

> The malignity of the contagion in this epidemic cannot be doubted; but the disease was often aggravated and made to assume its worst characters, by the most injudicious treatment. The prejudiced and most ignorant being the principal sufferers, the prescriptions of old women were more listened to than the advice of the medical attendant; a practice kept up by tradition amongst the poor was revived in spite of all remonstrance [...] 'At the commencement to set the object before a large fire and supply it plentifully with saffron and brandy to bring out the eruption; during the whole of the next stage to keep it in bed covered with flannel and even the bed-curtains pinned together to prevent a breath of air; to allow no change of linen for ten or more days until the eruption had turned; and to regard the best symptom to be a costive state of the bowels during the whole course of the disease [...]' The old nurses triumphed not a little in having an opportunity of showing their skill after it had been so long unexercised; nor was it often easy, amongst the deluded persons in whose families this affliction occurred, to persuade or compel them to adopt a different plan of treatment.[14]

As for preventing the spread of contagion, Crosse commented on 'the free intercourse which the children of the poor have with each other in a mild season, and the obstinacy of parents in voluntarily thrusting their children into danger which it was their duty to avoid'.

Inquiries made by Crosse and others showed much the same pattern being repeated in many rural districts. Amateur inoculation was rife, vaccination mistrusted, and the gleeful victory of the old women over the professionals in the matter of treatment, which must have been welcomed and encouraged by parents, testifies to the spirit of bloody-minded independence, however misguided, that prevailed at the time among the generally despised 'lower orders'.

CHAPTER 8

THE THREE BASHAWS

Even when the complex series of alliances and wars against the French ended with the final overthrow of Napoleon (an ardent admirer of Jenner), social unrest and the urgent need to contain it remained a constant preoccupation of successive governments. The year of the serious epidemic of smallpox in Norwich, 1819, was also the year of the Peterloo massacre in Manchester, with all that it implied for the current state of the nation, and there can be little doubt as to which event ranked as the more important in ministerial minds. During these years, when smallpox appeared, albeit slowly, to be loosening its grip on the population, apart from occasional displays of violence such as the epidemic that swept the country in 1825, the most insidious sickness affecting British society, more significant in its long-term effects perhaps than the electoral reform of 1832, was the steadily increasing growth of poverty. This was leading in many areas to chronic pauperism, especially in the southern agricultural counties, and a correspondingly increasing cost of trying to address this with an outmoded and creaking system of relief.

Random legislation first codified in late Elizabethan times prescribed measures for lightening the burden of the poor both on themselves and on their better-off compatriots. These had worked tolerably well for the better part of two centuries, but the stresses and upheaval created by the rapid evolution of an industrialized society, especially in rural communities, disrupted what had always been a somewhat uneven balance. By the 1820s the complaint heard in many quarters was that the national economy was in danger of collapsing beneath the burden of taxation in the form of poor rates levied on householders, which it was claimed were steadily reducing them to poverty themselves. The upshot, following the devastating report of the royal commission set up to investigate the situation, was the legislation known officially as the Poor Law Amendment Act of 1834 but popularly referred to as the New Poor Law. As with the report of the royal commission it was drafted almost entirely by the energetic reformer Edwin Chadwick and the radical economist Nassau Senior, who claimed to have written most of it himself. It does not call for detailed analysis here but certain of its major provisions need to be singled out.

Of the two kinds of assistance which, until the passing of the Act, had been at the disposal of local justices of the peace to be dispensed at their own discretion, the most frequently used and the most costly was outdoor relief in the form of payment in money or in kind. This was to cease immediately as being allegedly the source of much of the idleness, improvidence, profligacy and lack of independence that led the recipient down the road to pauperism and destitution and the ratepayers to potential bankruptcy. To reinforce the message, the alternative form of assistance, indoor relief, represented in the past by the offer of basic accommodation and the necessities of life in return for not-too-demanding labour, would in future be available to the able-bodied only if they accepted the 'workhouse test'. This required voluntary entry into a revamped institution to be conducted henceforth 'with the aim of making the indolent industrious', or, as a zealous reformer put it, 'to let the labourer find that the workhouse is the hardest taskmaster and the worst paymaster he can find and thus induce him to make his application to the parish his last and not his first recourse'. The corollary of this policy was the well-known principle of 'less eligibility' which laid down that no one inside the workhouse should at any time be better off than the poorest able-bodied labourer and his family outside it; life within its walls would of necessity be deliberately allowed to sink to such a level of deprivation that none but the most incorrigibly shameless would subject themselves to it.

As an integral part of the reorganization of the Poor Law the justices of the peace, stigmatized by Chadwick and Senior as the largely unwitting cause of the malfunctioning of the old regime because of their financial ineptness and insufficiency of rigour, were divested of all power over the administration of relief and replaced by a structure based on the amalgamation of parishes into 'unions' of appropriate size. In these all matters relating to the Poor Law were dealt with by boards of guardians elected by the ratepayers and operating under the general supervision of a Central Board consisting of three commissioners answerable, in effect, to no one but themselves.[1] The New Poor Law was established with little difficulty in the demoralized southern agricultural counties but met with fiercer resistance in the north where the tougher manufacturing class, more accustomed to the roller-coaster existence of booms and slumps, high wages and dire poverty, asserted their independence with the backing of a few enlightened employers and occasionally succeeded in disrupting the efforts of officials charged with establishing the statutory unions.

The practical consequences of transferring to elected guardians the responsibility for medical arrangements within their respective unions, with the avowed objective of curtailing expenditure in the interests of ratepayers, were soon apparent. In 1836 a meeting of the recently formed Provincial Medical and Surgical Association (PMSA), later to become the British Medical Association, drew up a petition addressed to both Houses of Parliament 'deprecating the system of medical relief adopted by the Poor Law authorities'. The petition dealt chiefly with the rôle of parish medical officers whose functions had been defined, with adaptations over the years, since Elizabethan times. Among its criticisms of the new system the petition complained that 'the greatly diminished and insufficient supply of medical officers must lead to the neglect and injury of the sick poor'; that 'the extent of medical districts [as necessitated by the new unions] in general precludes that prompt and convenient performance of medical duties which is essential to the proper treatment and safety of the sick paupers'; that 'the procuring of medical officers by public advertisement and "tender" (a practice degrading to the profession) is injurious to the public because it cannot afford a sufficient test of the qualifications and practical skill of the candidates'; that 'vesting in the hands of relieving officers the power of deciding whether the sick pauper required medical aid is calculated to prolong disease and endanger life'; and that

> entrusting to non-professional persons such as Poor Law Commissioners and Boards of Guardians the power of superintending and controlling, justifying and condemning, the conduct and proceedings of medical officers is neither just nor judicious and not in accordance with the practice pursued in other departments of the public service.

Unfortunately complaints based on comparisons with other 'departments of the public service' carried little weight at a time when the medical profession in general was still in a state of disorganization and internal rivalry, a situation that was not seriously addressed until the passing of the laboriously negotiated Medical Act of 1858. The anguished pleas on behalf of parish medical officers not only remained unanswered but were rendered more urgent still by a totally unforeseen development. In 1837 the first signs were noticed of the arrival of a strain of smallpox of an almost unprecedented ferocity, which gradually established itself nationwide, and was in Creighton's view 'one of the greatest [...] in the whole history of England'. From July 1837 until 31 December 1840 the epidemic smallpox in England and Wales caused 41,644 deaths, chiefly among infants and young children.

In 1840 the PMSA, meeting in Bath, adopted a proposal that a certain number of medical men should 'unite their labours in the investigation of the different branches of the subject of small-pox and vaccination'. A vaccination section chaired by Baron spent some time examining Jenner's disputed use of the words *'variolae vaccinae'* and ended by 'irresistibly proving his fundamental proposition, that Cow Pox and Small Pox are not *bona fide* dissimilar, but identical, and the vaccine disease is not the preventive of Small Pox, but the Small Pox itself, the virulent and contagious disease being a malignant variety'.

Turning from theoretical to practical matters the vaccination section made a number of proposals for improving the state of vaccination 'without interfering with prejudices which still unhappily stand in the way of more positive enactments [...] We propose [that] persons labouring under small-pox [should not] be exposed so as to disseminate disease [...] and only medical men be permitted to inoculate for small-pox'. An important step along a path stretching far ahead into uncharted territory was the proposal that

> duly qualified vaccinators should be appointed for every district in the kingdom, whose main duty should be, at certain seasons, to offer gratuitous vaccination to the poor of every hamlet and village or parish within their respective bounds. Stations and days and hours for vaccination might be fixed and also times for inspecting the progress of the affection. Registers, accurately constructed, would show every circumstance connected with perfect or imperfect vaccination...[2]

The petition also raised yet again the inadequate remuneration received by parish medical officers since boards of guardians had embarked so ruthlessly on their programmes of retrenchment.

The reference to registers was inspired by another recent legislative departure, the Registration Act which had come into force in 1837, setting up the Registrar General's department and requiring the obligatory registration of all marriages and deaths but not, for some reason, of births, which remained optional. The PMSA presumably envisaged the registration of vaccination details being undertaken by the officials who had been appointed under the Act, almost certainly without foreseeing how the process would get out of hand.

With surprising alacrity the government, roused from its customary apathy where smallpox was concerned, accepted a Bill under the title 'An Act to Extend the Practice of Vaccination', introduced in the House of Lords by the second Lord Ellenborough. The Bill was a short one but sowed the seeds of much discontent and controversy. Guardians and overseers of the poor were directed 'to contract with the medical officers of their several unions and parishes for the vaccination of all persons who may come to them for that purpose [...] Such medical officers shall make a report to the guardians and overseers of the number of persons then vaccinated.' Since one of the complaints of the PMSA was that there were already too few medical officers and in some areas none at all for the normal requirements of the sick poor, the imposition of a further burden in respect of vaccination did not augur well for the success of the new experiment. But the authors of the Bill had made provision for overcoming this obstacle: in any case where a medical officer was unwilling to take on further duties, 'it shall be lawful for the guardians to make [a] contract with any person not being a medical officer', with the proviso that this was an interim measure that would cease when a regular medical officer came along.

The Bill also made a half-hearted attempt to tackle the problem of inoculated smallpox:

> Any person not being qualified by law to practise as physician or apothecary, or not being a member of the Royal College of Surgeons, who shall inoculate with variolous matter for the purpose of causing the disease of the small-pox [...] shall be summarily proceeded against [...] and for every such offence shall be liable to be imprisoned in the common gaol or house of correction for a term not exceeding one month.

Inoculation was to be an offence only when performed by amateurs; it would remain legal for professionals.

The Bill provoked an immediate outcry on all sides, not for its specific proposals but for the concept of handing over responsibility for an important matter of public health to an organization set up to deal with destitution. Among the early protesters was H. W. Rumsey. In a letter addressed to the *London Medical Gazette*, written in April 1840 while the Bill was still passing through Parliament, he spoke of his astonishment that it had not 'already called forth a loud and general expression of disapprobation'. Recalling the suggestions put forward by the PMSA for 'a more universal and better regulated system' for the provision of vaccination he complained that, in attempting to promote the object of the petitioners, 'the legislature proposes to substitute a totally different machinery and to entrust poor law guardians and commissioners with the entire power of appointing public vaccinators, of determining their salaries, of regulating their proceedings and of inspecting their reports!' One of his specific criticisms was that, by entrusting vaccination solely to the Poor Law medical officers, 'the enactment is calculated in some localities to increase the prejudices against or indifference to this invaluable protection which are still too prevalent among the lower orders'. In other words, not even the offer of free vaccination, which they didn't set much store by, was likely to induce any self-respecting parent to have any truck with the petty tyrants who, wearing their Poor Law hats, ran the dreaded workhouse.

This was dramatically proved true a year or two later when the guardians of the parish of St George the Martyr in London announced that from a certain date all cases for vaccination must be performed at the workhouse. The Poor Law Commissioners, in a gentle remonstrance objecting to the arrangement, suggested that 'it would put an end to the general vaccination of residents in the parish, many of whom, not being paupers, would feel unwilling to take their children to the workhouse, under the impression that by doing so they were placing themselves in the position of paupers'.[3] The guardians ignored the warning and the number of vaccinations performed fell from 1,079 in the year before the decree to 42 in the year after it. Edward Seaton, in his *Handbook of Vaccination*, recalled that

> many of the local boards [...] saw in the proceeding little more than an additional burthen wantonly imposed upon 'the rates'. The names of those who had their children vaccinated were freely canvassed, and some boards went so far as to post on the church-doors the names of all who were vaccinated at the public cost, 'to shame them'.

Why had the government taken this unpopular and, to enlightened minds, retrograde step? In Rumsey's view it was the evident inclination of politicians 'to entrust all matters affecting the lives and health of the community to the discretion of a Malthusian board, a cause of painful apprehension to every humane and reflecting mind'[4] – a reference to the Reverend Thomas Malthus, whose notoriously pessimistic observations on the folly of trying to alleviate poverty among the feckless lower orders had profoundly influenced the begetters of the New Poor Law and their supporters.

Rumsey returned to the topic some years later in his *Essays on State Medicine*:

It matters not whether vaccination be termed a preventive or a palliative measure. Like all other public precautions against disease, it had been grievously neglected [...] The English Parliament resolved that something should be done; and as the poor-law machinery was ready at hand and willing to be worked our legislators deemed it quite needless to consider whether a more suitable machinery might not be desirable, or whether so unheard-of delegation of the sanitary functions of Government to a pauper-controlling department was at all consistent with sound political philosophy [...] In vain did physicians and surgeons throughout the land protest against the anomaly [...] the Poor Law Boards were appointed by a new law to direct (not the medical pauperization – be it observed, but) the vaccination of the whole working population.[5]

Apologists for the government claimed, and in some quarters still do, that it had no choice; the recently created Poor Law Commission was the first and still the only body operating nationally from a central base rather than through the piecemeal decisions of the 15,000 virtually autonomous parochial authorities that it had replaced: it would have been uneconomic, even if it had been feasible, to create a parallel organization to deal solely with vaccination. The opposing argument was set out in the *Lancet* in July 1848.

Vaccination is enforced and controlled in other countries by sanitary boards; but well-informed medical men are upon these boards [...] The degradation of being subjected to a poor law commission was reserved exclusively for the medical practitioners of England *because* they discovered and propagated the operation which other nations adopted.

This of course drew attention, not for the first time, to a second major consequence of the Act of 1840 – the hostility between the Poor Law Board, as it became, and the medical profession, which bedevilled relations between them for years to come.

Between the publication of the government's Bill in March 1840 and the completion of its passage through both Houses of Parliament, it underwent several changes, mostly designed to strengthen it. Fees payable for vaccinating the public free of charge 'shall depend on the number of persons who, not having previously been successfully vaccinated, shall be successfully vaccinated by the medical officer or practitioner so contracting', who was required to make a report to the guardians from time to time of the number of persons vaccinated. This was interpreted as an unacknowledged way of increasing the amount of vaccination by exerting pressure on the medical profession.

The supremacy of the Poor Law Commissioners was underlined by a requirement that they must be supplied with a copy of any contract entered into between a board of guardians and a medical practitioner. Any arrangement required for the execution of the Act must 'conform to regulations which from time to time may be issued by the Poor Law Commission'.

On the other hand two small concessions, the result of private initiative, were accepted by the government. In May, shortly before the Commons was due to take the report stage of the measure it was sponsoring, a Bill was announced 'to prevent inoculation for the small-pox and to extend the practice of vaccination'. The significance of this Bill in relation to the government's was twofold. It reversed the priorities by putting first the prohibition of inoculation for smallpox and making the ban total, with severe penalties for 'whomsoever shall produce or attempt to produce the disease of small-pox in any person'. Passing on to the question of vaccination it stipulated that when the operation was carried out on any person who had applied for it under the terms of the Act, 'no payment shall be made to any vaccinator who is not a legally qualified practitioner'.

The promoter of the Bill, Thomas Wakley, was a medical man of considerable stature, physical and intellectual, who has not found favour with some historians, perhaps because of his disruptive anti-establishment propensities. He qualified as a surgeon in 1817 and almost from the first set himself the task of limiting and, where possible, undermining the somewhat despotic power wielded by the autocrats of his profession as represented by the main corporate bodies, the Royal Society of Physicians, the Royal Society of Surgeons, who were for the most part at odds with each other, and the Society of Apothecaries. It was perhaps his swashbuckling, combative manner that earned him the disapproval of later commentators. To Creighton he was a radical whom the House of Commons, which he entered as the member for the large constituency of Finsbury in 1835, took seriously on medical matters 'if on no other', which does not wholly square with the reception given to his powerful speech, two and a half hours long, in defence of the Tolpuddle Martyrs, which led to a reprieve in 1836. A more recent author dismisses him as 'a violent, ill-tempered, somewhat eccentric radical doctor', which is simply a way of saying that he believed in making a nuisance of himself where complacent acceptance of the injustices of the status quo seemed to leave him no choice. An indication of the importance attached to medical expertise in those years is that he was the only member of the profession chosen to sit on the select committee which in 1839 looked into the working of the Poor Law Amendment Act. In the same year he took on the arduous post of coroner for West Middlesex. To Rumsey, who by no means despised him, it was to Wakley that 'the profession and the poor owed that fairer recognition of their claims and those admissions and recommendations which confirmed the truth of the chief complaints and the justice of the principal demands of the reformers'. Whatever view is taken of his campaigns and shortcomings he left one legacy that may be accepted as having lasting significance: in 1823 he founded the *Lancet*.

As a result of Wakley's intervention the Commons was faced in 1840 with two rival Bills on the subject of vaccination, one promoted by the government, the other the work of a notorious radical troublemaker. It could obviously not proceed with both and the outcome was predictable. Ellenborough's Bill became law, but with two less predictable but important concessions taken over from Wakley's: the total prohibition of inoculation for smallpox and an unequivocal acceptance of the principle that when appointing vaccinators, boards of guardians should negotiate not solely with their own medical officers but with 'any legally qualified medical practitioner or practitioners'.

Both victories were for the time being little more than symbolic. The whole complex problem of legal qualifications – who could claim them? who had the right to confer them? – had still to be thrashed out, and the stamping out of inoculation was far more easily decreed than achieved. Some distinguished authorities were opposed to the measure. Gregory, for example, pointed out that a child whose parents refused vaccination and who was now denied inoculation was in theory left with no protection at all from the casual disease, from which he concluded that since no parent in his senses would hesitate when such an alternative was placed before him, 'the whole population of England and Wales therefore are virtually by the Act compelled to submit to vaccination whether they like it or not'. In practice the problem was at this period unlikely to arise: in spite of Gregory's confident assurance that even in London the prohibition of inoculation was being 'rigidly enforced', the probability was that there would always be an unqualified but obliging quack or 'empiric' who, for a few pence and no questions asked, would slip round with some smallpox matter while the authorities were looking the other way and do the necessary.

Any satisfaction which the Poor Law authorities may have derived from their new status was soon overclouded by misunderstandings and objections to the procedure prescribed. 1840 was a testing time for the Commissioners. The select committee that had examined their performance since the passage of the Act of 1834 had received a great deal of criticism and complaint, including a long memorandum from a representative body of leaders of the medical profession. In accordance with the provisions of the Act the Commission would cease to exist at the end of the first session of Parliament held after 1839. The government had decided to introduce a Bill prolonging the life of the Commission for one year but the possibility was being canvassed that, in view of the contents of the select committee's report, it might change its mind. The Poor Law Commissioners' own report published in August 1840 was therefore an exceptionally lengthy and deferential document concerned chiefly with laying before the Home Secretary, Lord John Russell, 'those reasons in favour of the continuance of the Poor Law Commission which have not been adverted to by the Committee of the House'. It was particularly necessary that the Vaccination Act, which had come into force in the previous month, should be seen to be working satisfactorily. One week after the submission of their report to the Home Secretary the Commissioners issued an 'instructional letter' calling the attention of boards of guardians 'to the several provisions of the Act, with a view to the understanding of their object and the steps to be taken for their accomplishment'. The greater part of the circular consisted of a short induction course, of which many guardians were probably in need, on the necessity for preventing smallpox and the value and safety of cowpox inoculation, but one or two basic misconceptions, relegated to the final paragraphs, had also to be disposed of.

Hitherto, the letter explained, the guardians had had no power, nor had the Commissioners, to sanction any payment out of the rates for vaccination, otherwise than as medical relief in cases of destitution.[6] Under the terms of the latest Act guardians were directed to contract with medical practitioners in their several unions *for the vaccination of all persons resident in such unions* [...] [official italics]. The provision is now therefore legally extended to the whole population; to all those who are independent as well as those who are still dependent on relief or who may become so'.

No one can have viewed this development with greater disapproval than Edwin Chadwick who, expecting appointment as a Poor Law Commissioner, had been fobbed off with the far less distinguished post of Secretary to the Commission. What became of the principle of 'less eligibility' if the occupants of the workhouse could claim the same benefits, free of charge, as the respectable member of the middle class or the independent artisan? Boards of guardians had cause for dissatisfaction of a different kind. Entrusted with the welcome task of reducing the burden of the poor rates they had now somehow to fund the cost of medical attention, including payment to an additional layer of medical practitioners, for a service available, putatively, to every resident in their respective unions who cared to claim it. Some appear to have assumed, until reassured by the Commissioners, that the money would have to come out of their own pockets. Others could not believe that the law meant what it appeared to say. The Reform Act of 1832 stipulated that 'no person shall be entitled to be registered in any year as a voter in the election of a member of parliament [...] who shall within twelve calendar months [...] have received parochial relief or other alms'. The guardians in the Stamford union were of opinion, as they informed the Commissioners, that 'if parents who are voters voluntarily take their children to be vaccinated and suffer the fee of 1s. 6d. to be paid out of the poor rates it would be considered [...] under the Reform Act [...] as parochial relief, and would therefore, if objected to, disqualify them from voting'. In a lengthy reply the Commissioners informed the guardians of Stamford and other unions, who had apparently taken the same line, that they were wrong. Times had changed: the recent statute stated clearly that the right to free vaccination was neither 'relief' nor 'extraordinary relief'; it was extended to the whole population of England, Wales and Ireland, and it was as 'residents' that they received it.

It was obvious that the general indifference of the legislature to the problem of smallpox had allowed a thoroughly incompetent piece of drafting to pass into law, and within a year Parliament was called on again to try to restore order. In June 1841 the preamble to An Act to Amend an Act... casually and cordially admitted that in the statute of 1840, which was intended to extend the practice of vaccination, 'no express provision was thereby made defraying the expenses of carrying the same into execution', and that these could now be defrayed by guardians or overseers of the poor 'out of any rates or moneys which may come into their hands for the relief of the poor'. While they were at it the lawmakers took the opportunity to reiterate for the benefit of doubters that vaccination of any person or any member of his family should not be considered parochial relief, nor deprive any vaccinated person of 'any right or privilege, or subject them to any disability or disqualification whatever'.

Having got these misunderstandings straightened out the government handed the whole conduct of vaccination over to 'the three Bashaws of Somerset House', as they later became known, and got on with more important matters. This left the battle lines to be drawn for years of wrangling between guardians using every means to get vaccinators on the cheap, outraged medical men rejecting contracts on the insulting terms offered them, less scrupulous operators taking any terms they could get, and the Poor Law Commissioners trying tactfully to implant the notion that these manoeuvres would not in the long or even the short run provide guardians with the flow and quality of medical attention needed if they were to carry out their obligations as defined by the Act.

The severe smallpox epidemic of 1837–40 had been sweeping across the country and much of Europe. In November 1840, reflecting the degree of public consternation at all levels that had probably played a part in stirring the government into some show of activity, the *Lancet* carried a 'Note on the Present Epidemic of Small-pox and the Necessity of Arresting its Ravages'. The author, William Farr, was a mathematician and civil servant recently appointed to the General Register Office set up by the Registration Act that came into force in 1837.

Throughout his forty years' service, first as compiler of abstracts and later as superintendent of statistics, the 'Letter to the Registrar General' that he contributed regularly to the department's annual report provided unsurpassed insights into the nature of disease in general and the state of the public health. The opening words of his letter in the first annual report set out very clearly the wide scope and significance of his responsibilities as he perceived them:

> The deaths and causes of death are scientific facts which admit of numerical analysis; and science has nothing to offer more inviting in speculation than the laws of vitality, the variation of those laws in the two sexes at different ages, and the influence of civilization, occupation, locality, seasons, and other physical agencies either in generating diseases and inducing death or in improving the public health.[7]

At a time when civil servants appear to have enjoyed considerable freedom to express their own views and even to criticize their superiors, Farr's 'Note on Small-pox' displays an astonishing depth of passion and indignation and deserves lengthy quotation. His main concern was the situation in London. The prospect facing the city was the deaths of hundreds, possibly thousands of children from smallpox, and the fatality might be prevented by means of a discovery made by Jenner at the end of the previous century. If every unvaccinated person in the metropolis were vaccinated *during the next week* the epidemic would be arrested:

Is not a case for public interference, then, clearly made? Should not an energetic effort be made to save these lives, amounting to several thousands, from small-pox? They are helpless children, the great majority of them have not numbered 15 years […] They are in many cases the offspring of the poor, which again gives them a stronger claim on the humanity, justice and protection of society. Five children at the very least are destroyed daily by small-pox […] vary the statement slightly, and what would be the effect of the announcement in the *Times* or the *Morning Chronicle*: 'five children will be thrown from London Bridge daily during next week – the next twelve months – and the number will be raised to six, seven and eight daily in the next season'. The very supposition is revolting. Yet it gives but a fair idea of the reality. With the facts before them the people of this country can come to but one conclusion, that the entire population should be forthwith vaccinated…[8]

Farr claimed that the legislature had recently 'emphatically asserted the principle', but that the Act had not worked well, perhaps, he conceded, because it had not had a fair trial, and in a passage of slightly tangled syntax he seemed to distribute the blame for the failure between the Poor Law Commissioners for offering inadequate remuneration to vaccinators and the medical practitioners for refusing to accept it. The Bashaws, as might be expected, laid the blame elsewhere: 'From ignorance, indolence and their habits of procrastination, and carelessness about their offspring, and sometimes from the influences of quacks, the more pauperized classes have not brought their children to be vaccinated'. So how were they to be persuaded to do so? Could they – should they – be compelled to do so?

CHAPTER 9

A COMPETENT AND ENERGETIC OFFICER

For many years isolated voices had been hinting, some more discreetly than others, at the need for some kind of state intervention to enforce vaccination of the lower classes, but seldom using the blunt word 'compulsion'. The fear that inhibited stronger pressure was that enforcement might fail, not on medical but on political grounds. Warning that 'John Bull is jealous of the liberty of the subject', the *Lancet*, 'on the low ground of expediency, irrespective of right', called upon hasty legislators to pause. The legislators scarcely needed the warning: in spite of the manifest inadequacy of the Acts of 1840/41 no serious attempt was made for nearly a decade to pass beyond the voluntary principle into the dangerous waters of coercion.

Towards the middle of the century the balance decisively shifted. The medical profession, tired of having its hands tied by indifferent politicians and obstructive civil servants, turned from individual protest to concerted action. In September 1848 an anonymous letter to the *Lancet* urged the formation of a society for the study of the behaviour of epidemic disease. In July of the following year a public meeting, attended by 200 members of the medical profession and prominent figures from other walks of life, took place in Hanover Square under the presidency of the Earl of Shaftesbury, and the Epidemiological Society of London was inaugurated. The precisely stated objects of the Society were

> to institute a rigid examination into the causes and conditions which influence the origin, propagation, mitigation, prevention and treatment of epidemic diseases. It will be a part of the Society's province to ascertain the operation of existing enactments [and to] point out such alternatives as may be necessary for the protection of the public health [...] The Society propose to communicate with the Government and the Legislature in matters connected with the prevention of epidemic disease. [1]

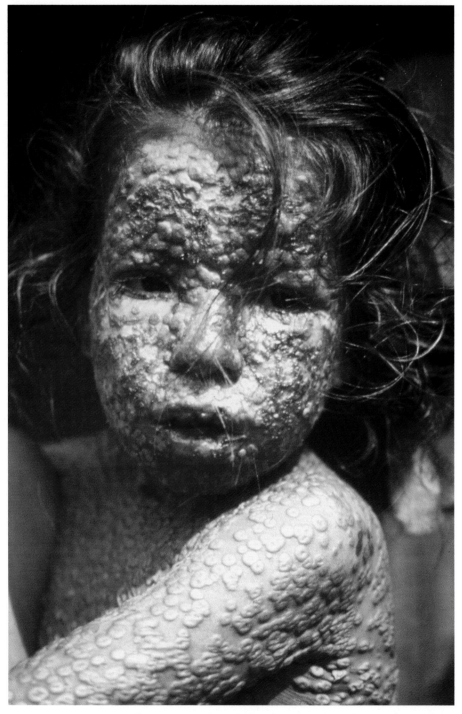

1. For centuries smallpox was one of the most feared diseases, not least because of the dreadful disfigurement suffered by those who survived an attack.

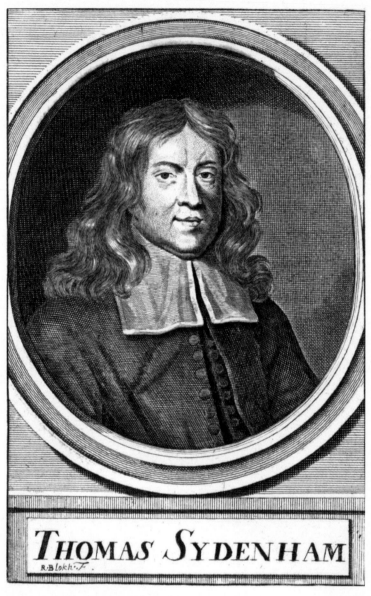

THOMAS SYDENHAM

2. Thomas Sydenham (1624–89), sometimes known as the father of English medicine, whose practice wih regard to the treatment of smallpox was based on clinical observation rather than theoretical abstraction

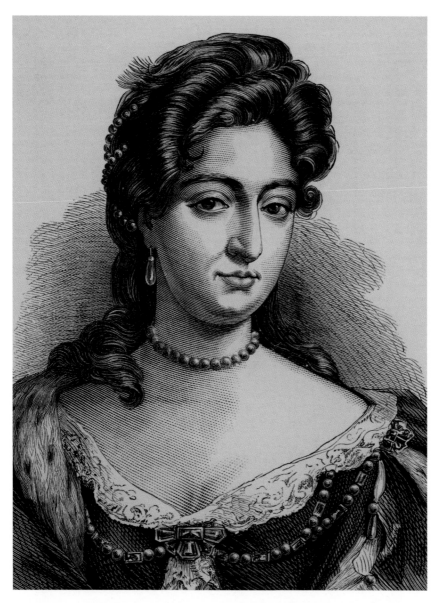

3. Although smallpox was prevalent among the poorest parts of society, the disease was no respecter of rank, and Queen Mary (1662–94) was its most notable victim, dying of the disease at the age of 32.

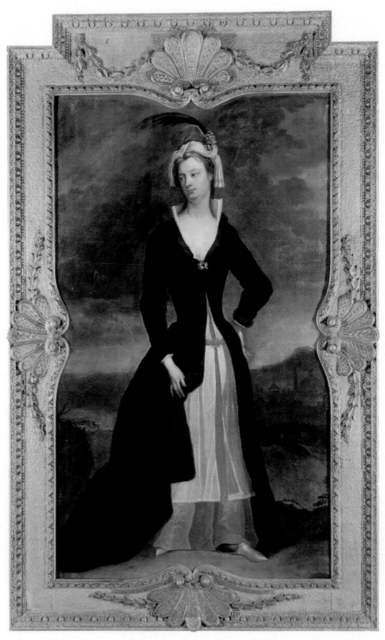

4. Lady Mary Wortley Montagu (1689–1762), here painted by Charles Jervas, is usually credited with bringing the practice of inoculation against smallpox into Britain, to be met with widespread hostility.

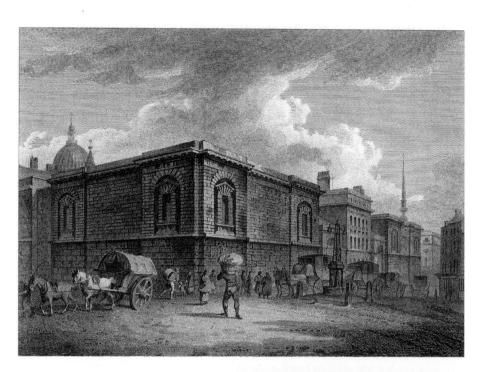

5. Newgate Gaol, the scene in 1721 of the first formal trial of inoculation, made under the direction of Sir Hans Sloane (1660–1753), the Royal Physician, with six volunteer prisoners as the guinea pigs. The trial was pronounced a success and led to a furthering of acceptance of the practice.

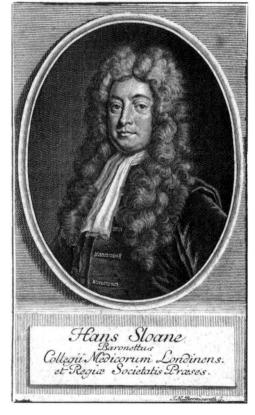

Hans Sloane
Baronettus
Collegii Medicorum Londinens.
et Regiæ Societatis Præses.

INSTRUCTIONS

FOR

The CONDUCT of PATIENTS under INOCULATION.

───◆───

OF PREPARATION.

THE following PREPARATORY DIET, beft fuited to the refpective age of the Patient, to be entered upon on the day of Inoculation.

For Breakfaſt.

Tea, with dry Toaſt; Milk Porridge; Skimmed Milk; Rice Milk; Panada; Water Gruel; Water Pap; Honey and Bread; or Bread made with the addition of Sugar and Currants.

For Dinner.

Bread Pudding; Rice or Millet Pudding; Plum or Plain Pudding; Apple Pudding; Panada; Milk Porridge; Rice Milk; and the production of the Kitchen Garden. Sugar, Salt and Vinegar are allowed with any of the foregoing articles.

For Supper.

A very fparing quantity of any of the above fpoon-meats; roaſted Apples or Potatoes.

For Children, a little weak Tea, or Milk and Water; with dry Toaſt, at an early hour (tea-time) is all that is requiſite.

As very little alteration can be made in the diet of young children, it is the more neceſſary, therefore, to render that which they are allowed to eat, as *thin* as can be difpenfed with, and that in fparing quantities. Children at the breaſt may be ftinted of that alfo, fhould it be required; but *Nurfes* themfelves need only abftain from high-feafoned inflammatory food and fpirituous liquors, and to keep their minds eafy as to the event.

Not allowed during Preparation.

Fiſh, Fleſh, Butter, Cheefe, Eggs, and Spiced Food, are not allowable at any meal. In fhort, whatever poffeffes a manifeſt heating quality, is improper during preparation; nor muſt the patient be indulged in eating between meals, unlefs it be *Fruits*, raw or prepared.

COMMON DRINK.

Toaſt and Water; thin Milk and Water; Barley Water; Imperial Water, or Lemonade. The patient muſt abftain from all fpirituous, vinous, malt liquors, and cyder: in fhort, whatever is drank, muſt be perfectly cooling; and, during the eruptive fever, a liberal ufe of them is generally neceſſary. The Small-Pox having made its appearance a few days, the patient may be indulged with a moderate quantity of wine and water, table beer, &c.

ALTERATIVE

6. A page from Daniel Sutton's *The Inoculator*, detailing part of the regime to be undertaken by a prospective patient. Sutton (1735–1819) used a simplified method of inoculation developed by his father, and by the 1760s was inoculating patients on an industrial scale. (© Wellcome Library, London)

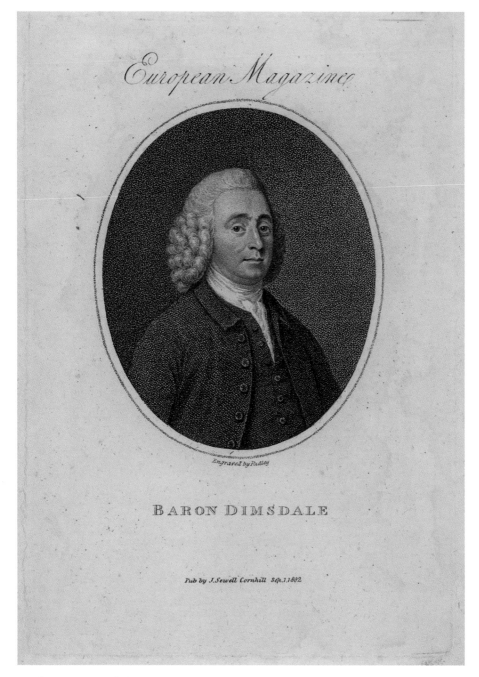

European Magazine

Engraved by Ridley

BARON DIMSDALE

Pub by J.Sewell Cornhill Sep.1.1802

7. Thomas Dimsdale (1712–1800), one of the most successful surgeons of his day, Physician to the Empress Catherine of Russia, and with Sutton, an enthusiast for mass inoculation.

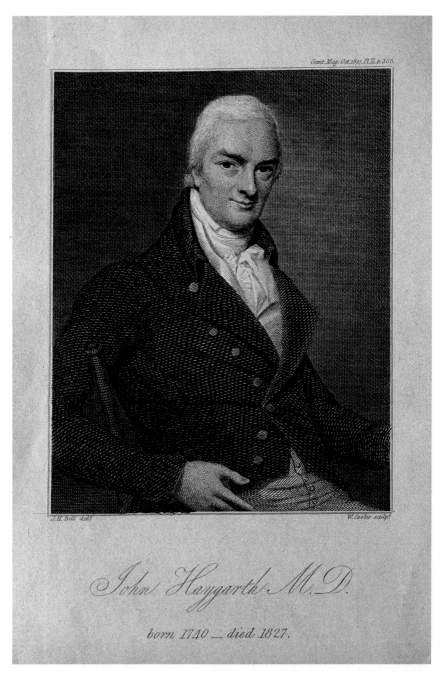

J.H. Bell del.   W. Cooke sculp.t

John Haygarth M.D.

born 1740 — died 1827.

8. John Haygarth (1740–1827) was one of the first medical practitioners to suggest that some form of legal compulsion might be necessary to ensure a sufficiently comprehensive take-up of inoculation against smallpox. (© Wellcome Library, London)

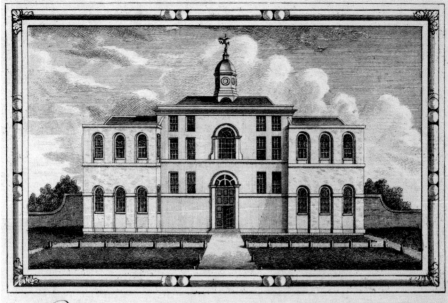

View of the SMALL-POX HOSPITAL near St Pancras.

9. The original Smallpox Hospital at St Pancras was opened in 1765 in one of the poorest areas of the city, much to the dismay of the local residents. In 1849 the Smallpox Hospital was moved to new premises on Highgate Hill as the site at St Pancras had been sold to make way for King's Cross railway station.

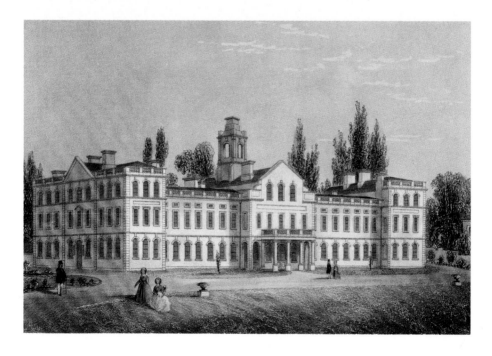

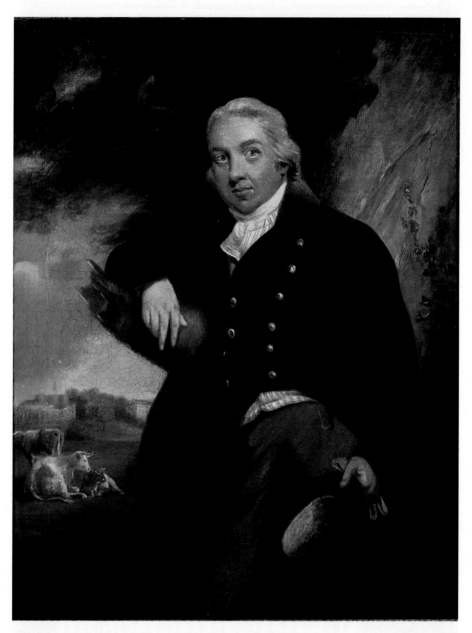

10. The popular impression that Edward Jenner (1749–1823) 'discovered' vaccination is inaccurate, but it is true that his investigation of the properties of cowpox and his advocacy were largely responsible for its adoption by the medical profession as a prophylactic against smallpox during the greater part of the nineteenth century. (© Wellcome Library, London)

AN

INQUIRY

INTO

THE CAUSES AND EFFECTS

OF

THE VARIOLÆ VACCINÆ,

A DISEASE

DISCOVERED IN SOME OF THE WESTERN COUNTIES OF ENGLAND,

PARTICULARLY

GLOUCESTERSHIRE,

AND KNOWN BY THE NAME OF

THE COW POX.

———

BY EDWARD JENNER, M.D. F.R.S. &c.

———

——— QUID NOBIS CERTIUS IPSIS
SENSIBUS ESSE POTEST, QUO VERA AC FALSA NOTEMUS.

LUCRETIUS.

———

London:

PRINTED, FOR THE AUTHOR,

BY SAMPSON LOW, N°. 7, BERWICK STREET, SOHO:

AND SOLD BY LAW, AVE-MARIA LANE; AND MURRAY AND HIGHLEY, FLEET STREET.

———

1798.

11. The title page of Jenner's *Inquiry,* published in 1798, in which he set forth his ideas about the relationship between cowpox and smallpox.

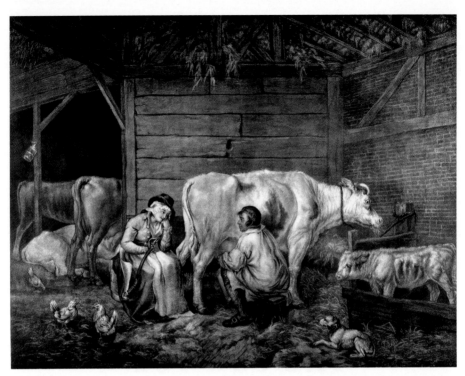

12. The common observation that milkmaids who had contracted cowpox from working in milking parlours became immune to smallpox led Jenner to the idea of deliberately infecting patients with the lesser disease so as to protect them against the more severe disease.

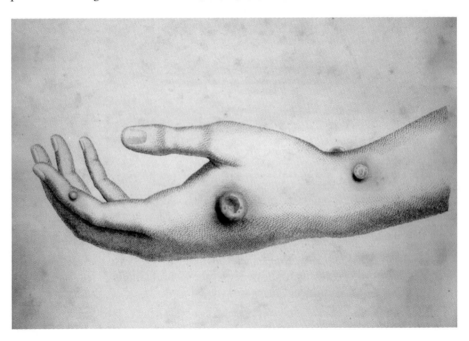

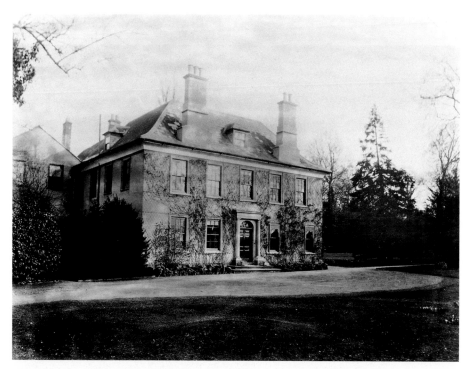

13. Jenner's house, The Chantry in Berkeley in Gloucestershire, which he bought in 1785, and the rustic hut in the garden, called by Jenner the Temple of Vaccinia, where he vaccinated his neighbours. (© Wellcome Library, London)

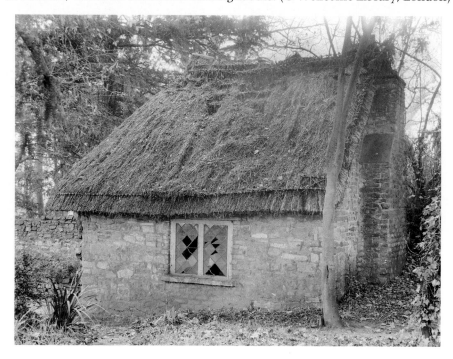

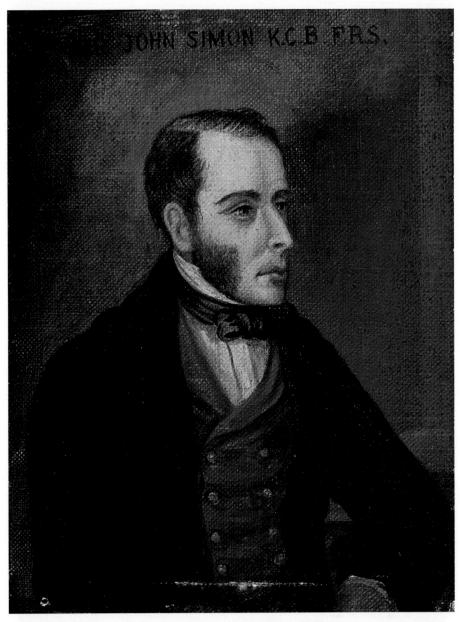

JOHN SIMON K.C.B F.R.S.

14. Following the introduction of the first Act to make vaccination compulsory in 1853, John Simon (1816–1904) was appointed as Chief Medical Officer to the Privy Council to take charge of a programme of systematic smallpox vaccination, a task which was made difficult both by the imprecision of the Act and the inadequacies of the vaccinators. (© Wellcome Library, London)

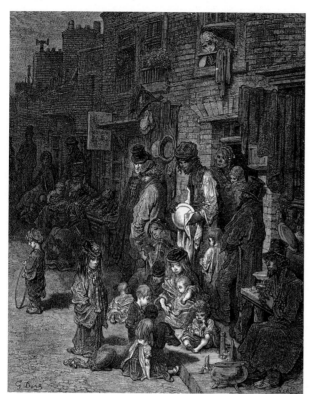

15. Gustave Doré's engraving of Wentworth Street, Whitechapel (1872) is a sobering image of the overcrowded and insanitary conditions that could accelerate the spread of disease.

16. This image from the *Graphic* of 1871 showing a public vaccinator at work in London's East End gives some idea of the chaos in which such practitioners were working, and might explain the reluctance of many to submit to compulsory vaccination. (© Getty Images, Hulton Collection)

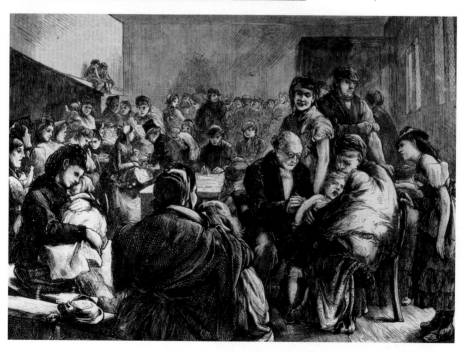

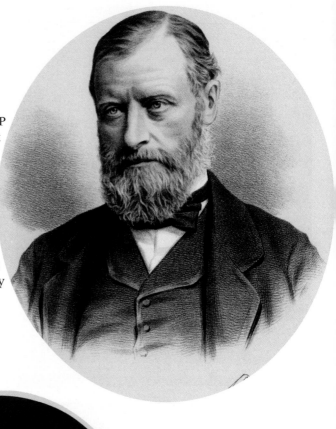

17. W. E. Forster (1818–86), MP for Bradford, chaired the select committee that considered the operation of the 1867 Vaccination Act, a contentious piece of legislation which caused widespread disquiet because of the draconian penalties it imposed on those who did not comply with its requirement for compulsory vaccination.

18. W. J. Collins, an anti-vaccinationist and member of the Royal College of Surgeons, sat on the Royal Commission that was set up in 1889 to consider the whole question of vaccination and compulsion. The Commission's recommendation that conscientious objectors to compulsory vaccination should not be prosecuted signalled a change in the official view of the desirability and efficacy of compulsion.

Numerous committees were set up to investigate subjects ranging from cholera to 'disease appertaining to the Vegetable Kingdom' and 'the question of supplying the labouring classes with Nurses in Epidemic and other Diseases', but there can be little doubt that the topic of immediate concern was the province of the 'Committee on Small-Pox and Vaccination'. The *Commemorative Volume* of the Society, published to mark its fiftieth anniversary in 1900, describes the efforts of this committee as 'almost epoch-making'. The attention of the Society was, from its earliest days, 'turned towards bringing about such legislation as would tend to reduce the heavy death toll (some 5,000 deaths yearly) from Small-pox'. Notice was formally served on the government that temporizing with the problem was no longer acceptable: nothing short of effective legislation would do, and the essence of the legislation that powerful members of the medical profession had in mind would almost certainly favour compulsion.

The committee laboured for more than two years assembling information and canvassing the opinions of '200 medical men practising in the United Kingdom and the British Empire'. The result of its efforts was a *Report on the State of Small Pox and Vaccination in England and Wales and on Compulsory Vaccination*, drafted almost certainly by the committee's secretary, Edward Seaton, and presented to the President and Council of the Society in March 1853.[2] The report necessarily covered in detail much ground familiar to students of the general problem, and tactfully paid compliments, which some may have considered rather over the top, to the Poor Law Board for 'the great anxiety of that body to secure the blessings of vaccination to the population [and] to express our conviction that no efforts have been spared to give efficiency to the [1840/41] Acts of Parliament'.

The fact had nevertheless to be faced that there were grave deficiencies, most of them inherent in the operation of the Act. The remuneration offered to vaccinators was in many cases 'pitiful'; even when the accepted going rate of 1*s.* 6*d.* for each vaccination was paid many public vaccinators deemed it too low and vaccination was often delayed until a large number of cases had accumulated, or until small-pox had broken out in the locality, 'a mode of procedure which it is obvious must often lead to sacrifice of life'; and there were boards of guardians who remonstrated whenever any large number of vaccinations had been reported. All of these factors had 'a tendency to check the efforts of medical officers, and thus to act prejudicially on the public welfare'. A long analysis of such reliable statistics as were available led to the conclusion that the annual average of cases of smallpox in the United Kingdom would not fall short of 100,000. 'Such is the humiliating

result of our own apathy 50 years after the discovery of vaccination.'
By contrast in most other countries in Europe, 'with or without the aid
of laws rendering the omission of vaccination penal the performance of
that operation is made essential to the enjoyment of so many munic-
ipal and other advantages that the general diffusion of it is pretty
certainly attained'. And no wonder: in Bavaria and France, for
example, 'even the rite of matrimony is withheld until the proper
certificates or other evidence of vaccination have been produced'. In
Austria there was no fine, 'but if it be known to the police that a person
is unvaccinated they have authority to take him forthwith and see that
the operation is performed'.

So to the verdict that had been implicit in the report from its opening
paragraphs:

> We desire [...] to state it as our unanimous conclusion [...] that no
> measure which does not render vaccination compulsory, in some
> form or other, will be sufficient to ensure the efficient protection
> of the population of this country from the ravages of small-pox.
> The mode of rendering vaccination compulsory it must be for the
> Legislature to determine: but in the event of its being deemed
> desirable to introduce a system of fines, we would suggest that the
> commencing fine be a small one, and that it be augmented from
> time to time until the requirements of the Act be complied with.[3]

A copy of the Society's report, forwarded to the Home Secretary, was
ordered to be printed by both Houses of Parliament and within a few
weeks preparations were being made for a Bill which would embody
most of its recommendations. There was some preliminary anxiety lest
it should be upstaged by a private initiative that had already been
making progress. Lord Lyttleton, a member of the House of Lords and
chairman of a board of guardians, had independently come to the same
conclusions as the Epidemiological Society and had drawn up, presumably with a little help from his friends, a Bill that he intended to bring
forward himself for the introduction of compulsory vaccination for
smallpox. The exact terms of his Bill seem not to have survived but
some of its provisions were generally held to be ill-conceived, and its
proposed treatment of the medical profession aroused bitter hostility.
Tactful negotiations took place hurriedly behind the scenes with a view
to securing a more acceptable measure without giving offence, or
worse, stirring up stubborn opposition to change. The President of the
Society, accompanied by members of the smallpox committee, had an
audience with Lyttleton and Palmerston, the Home Secretary. The

Lancet understood that 'Lord Lyttleton is not only willing but anxious to be put in possession of the opinion of the medical profession and as much as possible to act on them'. The result, although still far from satisfactory to the Society or the *Lancet*, was hastily introduced in the Lords and equally hastily passed to the Commons. With hardly any discussion, without even the formality of a division in either House, it was placed on the statute book in August 1853 as An Act to Extend and Make Compulsory the Practices of Vaccination. This 'extraordinary piece of legislation', as one historian has called it, passed by Parliament 'somewhat indifferently', was the fore-runner of the more draconian Acts of 1867 and 1871, which remained in force until they were finally killed off by the National Health Insurance Act of 1946.

The basis of the Act was the so-called arm-to-arm method of transmitting cowpox material which had itself been developed from the original method of 'ingrafting' smallpox in Turkey in the time of Lady Mary Wortley Montagu. The brief summaries in the margins of the text outline the proposed arrangements:

Parishes or Unions to be divided into districts for the purpose of vaccination, and places appointed for [its] performance. Parents and guardians of children born after 1st August 1853 to have such children vaccinated within three or four months after birth.

Children to be taken for inspection by [the] medical officer on [the] eighth day after the operation.

Certificate of successful operation to be delivered.

From the children brought in on the eighth day after their own vaccination the public vaccinator would select one or two with the best vesicles, or sores, from which he would extract matter, or 'lymph', with which to perform the operation on the day's new arrivals. The eighth day was the latest by which, according to Jenner, vaccine lymph from a vesicle was suitable for use.

As under the Act of 1840, boards of guardians would enter into contracts with medical officers or practitioners of vaccination at agreed rates for the performance of the operation. Vaccination could be postponed beyond the specified time limit if, in the opinion of the medical officers, the child was unfit to undergo it, and abandoned altogether if, after repeated attempts, the child was deemed 'unsusceptible of the vaccine disease'. The registrar of births and deaths in each district was responsible for ensuring that parents presented their newborn children, issuing a certificate of successful vaccination and entering the details in a special registration book, for the satisfactory completion of which duties he was entitled to a payment of threepence per child. The penalty to be imposed on parents for failing to have their children vaccinated in accordance with the law was a sum not exceeding twenty shillings.

The Act as passed was almost immediately shown to be unworkable and drew condemnation from all sides. Two years later the Epidemiological Society returned to the attack with a further report to the President of the General Board of Health 'on a proper state provision for the prevention of small-pox and the extension of vaccination'.[4]

The report drew attention to 'the deficiencies of the Compulsory Act and the evils of the present system'. The Act applied only to children born in England and Wales after a certain date and did not extend to the whole population, nor to immigrants; it professed to punish disobedience by fine or imprisonment, yet there was no one specially charged with its execution, or with the duty to proceed against offenders. It did not provide an efficient or workable system of registration. The arrangements made for the appointment of medical men as vaccinators were in many respects unfair to the profession and affected their willingness to co-operate. Vaccination had many prejudices to encounter; stamping it with pauperism or giving it 'the semblance of an act of poor relief' merely added to the prejudice and had retarded its acceptance by the class it was aimed at (its purpose having been described unequivocally in section I as 'affording increased facilities for the vaccination of the poor').

The conclusion reached by the report was that no improvement could be expected

> unless there be some competent and energetic medical officer to harmonise the whole system [...] to examine continuously its working [...] and in cases where it is required, to enforce the law whether against those who refuse to submit to vaccination or against those who by travelling about and improperly exposing themselves [...] diffuse small-pox throughout the Kingdom.[5]

The almost immediate response to the Society's paper was the publication in July 1855 of a 'Bill to provide for the vaccination of the people of England and Wales'. With what appears to have been a lack of foresight in the light of a critical situation facing the General Board of Health, the Bill proposed that the public vaccinators should be placed under the control of the Board, which would have the power to appoint medical inspectors and 'any legally qualified medical practitioner' to be a public vaccinator. This was little more than a preamble to the main proposals of the Bill which were unfolded in a succession of paragraphs:

VII   The Medical Superintendent of Public Vaccination shall make all the provisions necessary to facilitate the general vaccination of the people...

VIII   Every adult person residing in England and Wales on [1 January 1856] who shall not already have been successfully vaccinated nor had small-pox shall within three months cause himself [or herself] to be vaccinated by some duly qualified medical practitioner or by a public vaccinator...

IX   Every adult person who, after [1 January 1856] shall come to reside in any part of England and Wales [...] shall within three months after his [or her] arrival etc [...] [A similar clause had formed part of Lord Lyttleton's bill but had been withdrawn.]

As under the Act of 1853 the parent of any child 'who shall not have been successfully vaccinated' was given three months in which to have the operation performed; this applied to any child brought into the country from abroad. The sub-registrar who registered the birth of a child must 'deliver to the person attending' a notice that it was the duty of the parent to have the child vaccinated, and 'the non-receipt of such notice from the sub-registrar cannot be pleaded as a defence in any prosecution for penalties under this Act'.

This Bill was, not surprisingly, withdrawn. The much criticized Act of 1853 had failed because the administrative structure it relied on for its enforcement was too cumbersome and would have collapsed utterly under the additional strains to which the new Bill proposed to subject it. Moreover, even a body of legislators for the most part indifferent to vaccination must surely have baulked at the notion of requiring the whole adult population and every prospective immigrant to submit themselves and their children of whatever age to being vaccinated. Compulsion was all very well where children were concerned, especially those of 'the class it was aimed at'. The 'general vaccination of the people', however desirable in the eyes of the mandarins of the Epidemiological Society, was simply a non-starter; and perhaps the strangest aspect of the proposal was that none of them apparently perceived that it would be. The only significance of the Bill was that it represented the first and last attempt to secure the compulsory vaccination of the entire population of the country.

The matter was not destined to be put to the test. The Bill's proposals concerning the General Board of Health were rendered obsolete almost as soon as they were published by a strong turbulence that was currently buffeting the Board, largely as a result of the unpopularity of Edwin Chadwick, who had brought to his conduct of its affairs much of the autocratic intolerance and capacity to inspire hatred that had distinguished his handling of the Poor Law. By 1854 it had become obvious that nothing short of his removal would satisfy his enemies. An Act of that year provided that the General Board of Health should 'cease and determine' and be replaced by a new Board, whose members would consist of a President responsible to Parliament, which the old Board had lacked, and the principal secretaries of state of the Committee of Council 'appointed for the consideration of matters relating to Trade and Foreign Plantations'.

Unfortunately the passions aroused by the Chadwick era had reached too high a level to be easily assuaged. The new Board's existence was limited to one year, and was subsequently renewed on an annual basis until a return to normality in 1859. The most significant step forward during this period of upheaval was the permission granted by the Continuance Act of 1855 for the appointment by the Board of 'a Medical Council [...] and a medical officer with salary and travelling and other expenses'. This left the way clear for the realization of the Epidemiological Society's demand for 'a competent and energetic officer to take charge of vaccination'. The man chosen was John (later Sir John) Simon. One of the founders of the Society and a member of the council, a distinguished surgeon at St Thomas's Hospital, a post he continued to occupy in addition to his new appointment, he had worked closely with Chadwick and gained a high reputation as the first medical officer of health for London.

The timing of his appointment could hardly have been less auspicious, with his new employer, the General Board of Health, limping along to almost certain extinction, at least in its present form; existing, as Simon put it, 'only provisionally – it had no settled structure or vocation of its own'. This was not what he had expected or hoped for: 'the position in itself soon became humiliating. To "stand and wait" in the ante-chamber of legislation was not to "serve" in the sense of Milton's great verse.'

This, however, is not the whole story. In his own account of the next four years or so Simon conveys the impression that nothing of importance happened, at least as far as he was concerned: 'A limited amount of business was carried on [...] To dwell at large on that business would not now [1890] be of interest.'[6] His biographer paints a different picture: 'Simon's arrival at the Board of Health transferred the reforming principle into administration. He quickly shaped the [Epidemiological] Society's proposals into Government Bills [...] introduced in 1856 and 1857'.[7]

The Bill of 1856 proposed to 'consolidate the law relating to vaccination', and would have repealed all previous Acts, while leaving contracts already entered into to continue. The main provisions of earlier Acts would have been retained but with significant additions. Clause 12 would have brought private vaccinators within the scope of the Act: 'Managing committees of schools receiving aid from government grants, the masters of workhouses, the keepers of lunatic asylums and governors of prisons' would be able to inquire into the vaccination of children attending or incarcerated in these institutions and 'direct the vaccination of all such persons as they find unvaccinated'. A new departure would have empowered coroners to hold inquests on unvaccinated children who died of smallpox. The penalty for not having a child vaccinated remained a maximum of twenty shillings and in the case of a continuing refusal or neglect, a penalty would be imposed not exceeding five shillings 'for every day during which such neglect shall be continued from and after receipt of any notice from a guardian or overseer'.

When the Bill came before the Commons in March 1856 it met with a largely hostile reception. Criticism centred on its failure to deal with the problem of dual control shared between the General Board of Health and the Poor Law Board, on reports of adverse comments from parents concerning the ill effects that vaccination was allegedly having on children, and on the whole purpose and compulsory apparatus of the Bill in its entirety. Parliament had no right, one dedicated opponent maintained, to authorize the General Board of Health to go into a man's house and say to him, 'You shall submit to have a disease conveyed to you which may imperil your life'.

The expression of anti-vaccinationist sentiment had still to take a concerted form, but this warning of possible rough seas ahead clearly alarmed the government. The Bill was read a second time and then disappeared from view for so long that Thomas Duncombe, a member notorious as a professional thorn in the side of governments, asked for news of it. Cowper[8] replied maladroitly that the Bill was not one in which members usually took a great interest. It was one of that class of Bills which were usually taken at a late period of the evening. He hoped the honourable member would not object to this course being followed. This was not unnaturally taken as an indication that the government, aware that it had an unsatisfactory and unpropitious measure on its hands, had been caught trying to slip it past the House when virtually no one would be paying attention. Duncombe disabused the minister: it was a 'compulsory bill': 200 petitions had been presented against it and only one in its favour. 'A more arrogant job than this bill I never knew and I hope I may be given an opportunity to oppose it.'

Cowper replied weakly to the effect that if Duncombe felt like that it would be fairer if he brought in a Bill to repeal compulsion (Duncombe later took him at his word with a Bill to repeal the Act of 1853 on the ground that it was 'inexpedient' to enforce it), but in the present circumstances he, the minister, promised not to bring the Bill in after midnight.

It reappeared a few weeks later, much amended and emasculated to the point where the life had gone out of it. Hardly anyone had a good word to say for it. Duncombe, recalling that the 1853 Act had been 'smuggled through the House at a late stage in the session', admitted to a belief that 'great good had resulted from vaccination', but he did not think it would be encouraged by penal enactment.

Cowper took the view that the opposition that had been shown was directed more against vaccination than against the Bill, and went on to make an admission which put the whole exercise in perspective. It might be that there was something in the manner in which vaccination was performed among the poorer classes that prevented its being as safe and efficient a precaution as it was for the richer portion of the community; '[t]hey were not however legislating for the higher but for the lower classes.' He therefore proposed to adopt a suggestion from Dunscombe that the Bill be discharged (i.e. not proceeded with) and that a select committee of the House be appointed in the next session 'to look into the manner in which vaccination was performed in practice'.

Whatever part Simon had played in this fiasco – certainly the Bill as drafted incorporated elements symptomatic of his thinking and that of his future right-hand man, Seaton – his first foray in 'the ante-chambers of legislation' had proved unpromising and it is not surprising that thirty-five years later he preferred not to recall it. The immediate consequences were in fact less disadvantageous to him than might at first have been expected. According to a *Historical note on the Prevention of Smallpox*,[9] written by a Ministry of Health official years later, it was as a direct result of the paper prepared by the Epidemiological Society in 1855 that the President of the General Board of Health had requested Simon to lay before him 'such evidence as will assist him in estimating the hygienic value of vaccination and the strength of any objection which have been alleged against its adoption'. Simon offers a different account of the sequence of events. Describing the withdrawal of the Bill of 1856 he makes no mention of a specific request from Cowper but stresses his duty to prepare himself as thoroughly as he could for the promised select committee, by reducing into convenient form 'the vast quantities of evidence available'. The select committee followed the Bill into oblivion, but 'fortunately the then circumstances of the Board' (presumably its imminent demise) 'allowed me to undertake the task on a far larger scale than would [otherwise] have been possible'. The result, presented to Parliament in July 1857, was *Papers Relating to the History and Practice of Vaccination*, which became known simply as *Vaccination Papers*, attracting widespread attention and referred to for years to come as the 'bible' on the subject. The verdict of Simon's biographer may be quoted: 'The *Papers* were exhaustive in treatment, monumental in their conclusiveness and comprehensive in their scope, representing, as the author said, "the experience of the civilised world as to the use of vaccination".' Modern scientists, Lambert concedes, would not go along with some of the positions Simon adopted but 'they would wholly endorse his conclusion: "Jenner's discovery – properly utilised – has been a blessing to mankind, an unmixed addition to the strength and happiness of nations".'[10]

Simon's own considered estimate of his achievement was more modest:

> Looking back from [a] distance of thirty-three years [...] I of course find passages which I would wish amended. Especially I observe that, here and there, entering needlessly on questions of speculative pathology, I slid into more *a priori* reasoning than I should in later years have deemed suitable to the matter; and in respect of some such passages I could now amend my arguments by later knowledge. In more general respects the Report is mainly a compilation of facts: in which sense I trust it may prove useful.[11]

The questions posed and answered in the *Papers*, as summarized by Simon, were essentially those that would have naturally followed from the request allegedly made to him by Cowper:

1) What kind of an evil was smallpox before vaccination arose to resist it?

2) What facts and arguments led to the first sanction of vaccination and to what sort of inquiry were they subjected?

3) What further knowledge, at the end of half a century's experiment, have been gathered on the protective powers of vaccination?

4) What evils have been shown to attend its practice, and to counter-balance its advantages?

5) How far are there realized, in this country, those benefits that can reasonably be expected from a general use of vaccination?

The pages of the *Papers* dealing with the early history of vaccination appear to be heavily indebted to Baron in their unrestrained enthusiasm for Jenner and their somewhat uncritical account of his 'discovery', a word already deprecated in most quarters, even by 1857. The words of 'the dairy-folks of Gloucestershire', once spoken in Jenner's hearing, were 'never afterwards absent from his mind. Thirty years elapsed before their fruit was borne to the public, but incessantly he thought, and watched and experimented on the subject' the result emerging as 'that masterpiece of medical induction', demonstrating 'the patience and caution and modesty with which Jenner laid the foundation of every statement he advanced'. The *Inquiry* 'cited in detail many instances of persons who, having at earlier periods of life accidentally contracted an infection from cows or horses, had afterwards shown themselves insusceptible of human small-pox'. The instances included 'twenty-three cases in which by vaccination the human system had been rendered, for periods ranging up to 53 years insusceptible of small-pox inoculation'.

The extent and quality of Jenner's research came in for scathing criticism later in the century, and no one relying on Simon's narrative (as most of his contemporaries would have done) would have been aware that the first version of the *Inquiry*, intended for publication by the Royal Society, was not thought worthy of acceptance; a further indication perhaps of Simon's reliance on Baron, who was himself accused years later of having deliberately misled his readers by making no reference to this embarrassing episode.

After this somewhat ill-considered beginning the *Papers* settle down into a more straightforward account of the development of Jenner's ideas and the contribution made by his contemporaries. It was perhaps surprising that even at that date, in spite of doubts and ostensibly reliable evidence assembled over a period of fifty or more years, Simon was prepared to assert, with only a perfunctory nod in the direction of revaccination at the period of puberty, that vaccination performed in infancy in the best manner gave to most persons through life a complete security against attacks of smallpox.

One source of which he made much use, reprinting it among other documents at the end of his own *Papers,* was a petition on the Vaccination Bill of 1856 addressed to 'the Honourable the Commons of the United Kingdom of Great Britain and Ireland, in Parliament assembled' (possibly the 'only one in favour' mentioned by Duncombe). The author was James Marson, for twenty years the resident surgeon at the Smallpox and Vaccination Hospitals in London, where he claimed to have attended nearly 9,000 cases of smallpox and vaccinated upwards of 40,000 persons. His petition was in effect a defence of the operation and a plea for the better performance of it. The mortality of smallpox in the unvaccinated, taken generally, was 35 per cent, but of children under five years of age it was 51 per cent, and of those who recovered a great many suffered a permanent disfigurement and even worse disabilities. The mortality among the vaccinated attacked by smallpox was 7 per cent, taken generally: among the well-vaccinated only one-third of 1 per cent. Among children under fourteen who had been vaccinated smallpox hardly ever proved fatal: the badly vaccinated suffered after-effects almost as grievous as the unvaccinated.

The reality that Marson had clearly wished to impress upon the legislators, and particularly the timid ministers who were about to sell the pass by abandoning the Bill currently before Parliament, was that 'no authorized system of vaccination has been established in England'. The result, frequently adverted to over the years, was here spelt out again by Marson, in uncharacteristically vivid language:

> All persons – medical men, clergymen, amateurs, druggists, old women, midwives, etc. – are allowed to vaccinate in any way he or she may think proper, and the persons operated on are considered to have been vaccinated. The consequence of this carelessness and want of arrangement is, that there has been, and is, a great deal of very inefficient, almost useless vaccination performed in England.[12]

This was the situation three years after the Act of 1853 had made vaccination compulsory. Not the least important conclusion to be drawn was that pretty well all statistics quoted in any quarter since Jenner had first vaccinated young Phipps were unreliable and could be consigned to the scrap-heap. A further inference was that parents who declined to submit their children to vaccination in the existing state of confusion might well have every justification for their stand.

These were among the issues that Simon addressed in the *Papers.* The recent Bill had been thrown out, in spite of Marson's earnest eloquence, because opponents in Parliament were making threatening noises. Opposition outside Parliament, although muted and sporadic, had been growing since the imposition of compulsion in 1853.

A letter of protest written in 1856 by one John Gibbs, effectively furnishing the text of forty years of bitter conflict, had so deeply impressed the recipient, Sir Bernard Hall, President of the Board of Health, that he caused it to be printed and circulated as a government paper, to the fury of the medical and political establishments, which were by now almost unanimously in favour of compulsion. Simon's *Papers*, issued a year later, were in effect if not wholly by design a riposte to Gibbs' letter; almost every subsequent utterance on the subject was derived ultimately from one or other of their basic positions. To Gibbs, compulsion in this sphere, as ordained by the Act, was a totally inadmissible infringement of the personal liberty of the subject; to Simon only those 'unacquainted with the circumstances under which the law was made' could have viewed it as 'an improper restriction on personal freedom'. The question was not whether people should be prevented from 'cultivating a personal taste for small-pox'; the object of the law was

> to prevent them from *compelling* (for in this case *allowing* amounts to *compelling*) their children to incur the worst perils of that disease [...] The practical justification of any such law depends on the amount of evil which it is designed to correct; and four or five thousand annual deaths by one specific parental omission constituted in this case a strong argument [...] It was this *liberty of omissional infanticide* which the law took courage to correct.[13]

While standing firmly by the policy of compulsion Simon candidly admitted, as he could hardly avoid doing in the light of Marson's testimony, that in one respect both the law and the practice were grossly unsatisfactory. If the state required some two thirds of the population to be compulsorily vaccinated it had a moral obligation to ensure that 'what it invites and compels people to accept shall be at least of good quality'. This, as things stood, it demonstrably was not. The law stipulated that only 'legally qualified medical practitioners' should be contracted as public vaccinators, but no one had so far succeeded in defining what, in this context, the phrase implied. In plain terms:

> a medical student may [...] obtain his diploma, license and degree [...] may become, in every possible sense of the words 'a legally qualified medical practitioner' – may be eligible and actually elected for the appointment of public vaccinator – and meanwhile

may never have performed, perhaps even never have witnessed, one single act of vaccination.[14]

This was one of the areas in which far-reaching reforms were required, and there was much work to be done before the terms of the necessary qualification could be agreed on and a programme of training implemented. For the time being Simon could do little except make preparations for the day when the conflict over the General Board of Health would be resolved. The existing stalemate could not be tolerated much longer, and clearly the unpopular and largely impotent Board of Health would have to go. The decisive step was an Act, passed in 1858, 'for vesting in the Privy Council certain powers for the protection of the public health'. As part of this reorganisation 'the person who at the time of the cessor of the General Board of Health may be their medical officer shall become the medical officer of the Privy Council', with a particular remit to improve the system and quality of vaccination. In this perhaps unlooked-for manner John Simon was released from the limbo in which he had languished for three years; but what, it might have been asked, qualified the Privy Council to assume responsibility for the health of the nation?

The functions of royalty by the middle of the nineteenth century were, in Bagehot's words, 'for the most part latent', and the functions of the Privy Council had largely followed them into a similar state, tending towards the dignified rather than the efficient parts of the constitution. Deprived of the power its members had once enjoyed as counsellors and brakes on the powers of monarchs the Council had dwindled, except as far as its judicial functions were concerned, into an advisory body discharging miscellaneous but useful functions, such as overseeing Trade and Foreign Plantations, for which no other machinery of government existed.

In the early part of the nineteenth century, for example, it had become clear that private charity was no longer providing adequately for the education of the labouring classes and that the state would have to contribute. In 1833 a grant of £20,000 was made 'in aid of private subscriptions for the erection of school houses for the education of the poorer classes in Great Britain'. By 1839 the sum involved had risen to £33,000 and, in the absence of anything remotely resembling a Ministry of Education, a committee of the Privy Council was set up to administer the fund under the stewardship of a secretary, John Kay-Shuttleworth. Once launched on this slope governments found there was no going back. More intervention was continually required to prop up the ailing voluntary system, more funds were voted until, with the grant running at nearly half a million pounds, the time had clearly arrived when Parliament must play a more active supervisory role, if only to ensure that the state was getting value for its money. In 1856 the Committee of Council was transformed into the Education Department and an official bearing the imposing title of Vice-President of the Committee of the Privy Council for Education was put in charge, with a seat in Parliament. This sequence of events created a precedent for further measures of a similar kind. The Public Health Act of 1858 stopped short of handing over to the Privy Council the supervision of all matters pertaining to the public health: some powers came to rest in the Home Office, and the ambiguous role of the Poor Law Board as the body responsible for overseeing the contractual arrangements for vaccination, with the Privy Council as the medical authority, was left untouched to muddy the waters for several decades to come.

The whole issue was still in fact in doubt. The vexatious Duncombe succeeded, with considerable backing, in causing this Act, like its predecessors, to be limited to one year only. When the question of renewal came up for consideration early in 1859 the state of the parties in Parliament was, in Simon's words, 'eminently not that in which Ministers are expected to stand by their proposals'. He was at one time given to understand that Lord Derby's administration, which itself had held office for little more than a year, proposed to let the Act lapse, and his appointment with it, but fortune was for once on his side: it was the administration whose life expired before that of the Act. As a result, it was alleged, of pressure from the Prince Consort behind the scenes, the incoming administration of Lord Palmerston was induced to stand by its predecessor's legislation. In July 1859 a Bill 'to make perpetual the Public Health Act, 1858' was steered through the Commons by the narrowest of margins on the third reading, and Simon's appointment was finally made secure.

The Act of 1858 had specified that the powers inherited by the Privy Council could be exercised by any three of the Lords, and other members, the recently appointed Vice-President of the Committee of Education being one of them; it was Robert Lowe, the current holder of the office, who had secured the latest and decisive victory. This yoking of education and vaccination, which had the appearance of an afterthought rather than a bold stroke of positive policy, points to what, to a later age, might appear something of a paradox but seems to have aroused no comment at the time. For a period in the mid-nineteenth century a parent was under no obligation whatever to have his offspring educated, but the state would fine him and in due course imprison him for neglecting or refusing to have them vaccinated.

CHAPTER 10

FORMIDABLE MEN

In his life of Leslie Stephen, *The Godless Victorian*, Noel Annan describes 'the new experts', the reformers and administrators who dominated and defined the emerging society of early and mid-Victorian Britain:

> They were men of inexhaustible energy, of disinterested probity, of indefatigable industry; but tact, compromise and suavity were foreign to their natures. They had the strength of mind to establish principles for dealing with the problems they were set, but once formed they could admit no other and closed their minds because the administrative structures they had invented seemed to them the only feasible way of dealing with the problem...[1]

The most obvious example of this breed of 'formidable men', as Annan calls them, was Edwin Chadwick, one of the principal architects of the New Poor Law of 1834. This had replaced a 'ramshackle and extravagant contrivance', but Chadwick remained impervious to the outcry that his reform was harsh and 'inhumane'. John Simon had worked with Chadwick as his 'noble disciple and friend', in the words of one commentator, and in his own study of *English Sanitary Institutions*, written when he was himself no longer playing an active part in public life, he went out of his way to defend Chadwick from some of the more severe charges levelled against him:

> In the earlier stages of Mr. Chadwick's career, when the essence of his work was to force public attention to the broad facts and consequences of a great public neglect, it mattered comparatively little whether, among his eminent qualities he possessed the quality of judicial patience; but in his subsequent position of authority demands for the exercise of that virtue were great and constant...[2]

Among the faults for which Chadwick was then criticized were 'a liability to one-sidedness on questions of science and administration, a failure to listen duly to dissentient voices [...] and a too despotic tone in affairs of local and personal interest'; but these might be generalized as 'faults of over-eagerness [that] fall into moral unimportance as compared with his sincere and disinterested zeal for the public service'. Confronted with evidence of unnecessary human suffering, 'the indignation which he was entitled to feel [...] is a not ignoble excuse for such signs of over-eagerness as he may have shown'.

The apologia is elegantly, even dispassionately expressed, but Simon seems to be putting in a plea in his own defence. Faced twenty or so years earlier by much needless human suffering caused by the failure to make the best use of vaccination in the battle against smallpox, he had responded in the same uncompromising spirit as Chadwick in similar circumstances. The course of the battle and the price of victory are described in Royston Lambert's standard biography of Simon, which appears to reveal a conflict, perhaps unconscious, in the biographer's mind between admiration for Simon's administrative machine for enforcing compulsion and an uneasy awareness of its unacceptable human consequences.

The vaccination system, Lambert writes, represented 'an extremely early development of state interference: a free, compulsory and national health service in miniature [that] deserves in many ways the pride of place of the pioneer'. The basis of the system (pre-dating Simon's involvement) was the Act of 1853 ('this extraordinary piece of legislation') by which 'somewhat indifferently Parliament had created a stringent, universal and utterly novel interference with human liberty'. A Bill that would have widened compulsory vaccination from newborn infants to the entire population 'unfortunately [...] met resistance from a nascent anti-vaccination movement now spreading in the country', and was dropped. But the 'pretensions' of the anti-vaccinationists were 'exploded' by Simon's *Vaccination Papers*, which, however, combined 'the experience of the civilised world as to the use of vaccination' with 'an imprecise understanding of the secondary dangers of vaccination'.

In 1857 Simon is seen to be advising that compulsion should not be 'applied in an oppressive, dogmatic manner', but following the passage of the Vaccination Act of 1867, with its 'astounding' clause 31 ('the most inhuman and severe in any health statute imposed upon the whole civilian population of England'), the powers taken by the law are being exercised with 'a stringency unprecedented in English health legislation'. By 1876 central control of vaccination has reached its *'nec plus ultra'* with its architect John Simon driven by 'empirical necessity and scientific convictions' to operate 'a refined machine of coercion unmatched elsewhere in the sanitary systems of this country or the world'. Lambert's conclusion is that it was 'all worthwhile'.

Somewhere along the route the assiduous reader of footnotes will discover that when giving evidence to the Royal Commission on Vaccination in 1889 Simon 'admitted the faults of the *Vaccination Papers*'[3] and that according to Lambert he was not 'aware of the grave secondary dangers involved in the method' of arm-to-arm vaccination which was the foundation of the entire edifice of compulsion until it was prohibited in 1898.[4]

The main outlines of the story can now be retraced in rather more detail and from a slightly different perspective. We have seen that Simon was at first, to some extent, impeded by Duncombe's success in delaying the renewal of the 1858 Act for one year, but once that obstacle had been removed the damage proved to be not too serious. The Act, as passed, gave Simon, on behalf of the Privy Council, powers sufficient to enable him to make a start on his programme of reform. Clause 2 empowered the Council to issue from time to time 'such regulations as they see fit for securing the due qualifications of persons to be hereafter contracted with by guardians and overseers [...] and for securing the efficient performance of vaccination'. It also brought the National Vaccine Establishment under the control of the Council. Clause 3 authorized the Council to cause to be made 'such inquiries as they see fit in relation to any matters concerning the public health in any place or places, and to the observance of any regulations and direction issued by them under this Act'.

Less successful, from Simon's point of view, was Clause 8, which broke new ground and must have contributed greatly to the reluctance of a significant section of the Commons to vote for the Act when it came up for renewal at the end of its stipulated year:

> Proceedings for penalties under these Acts [...] on the subject of vaccination may be taken on the complaint of any registrar [...] public vaccinator or officer authorised by the board of guardians or overseers respectively, and the cost of such proceedings shall be defrayed out of the common fund of the union [...]

It was at this period that the cause of vaccination suffered one of those vicissitudes to which it was so often subjected. A price of some kind had to be paid by Robert Lowe to buy off opposition to the renewal of the Act. Proclaiming himself 'no friend to compulsory vaccination', he dropped Clause 8, thereby depriving the reformers of one of their principal weapons. He later conceded that he had been ill-advised to sacrifice the clause and resurrected it by means of a separate Act three years later.

This hiccup at the start of their professional relationship must have seemed to Simon not to augur well for an untroubled collaboration between them, but in spite of it they worked harmoniously together, not only during Lowe's tenure of office as Vice-President, but also when he became Chancellor of the Exchequer, and Simon, as first holder of the post of Medical Officer, acknowledged his 'personal reason to feel indebted to Mr. Lowe for the sort of apprenticeship which my years of service under him afforded me'. The terms of the Act which transferred certain areas of public health to the Privy Council meant that for practical purposes the Vice-President *was* the Council, and this, combined with the virtual autonomy enjoyed by the Chief Medical Officer (as he ultimately became), made Lowe and Simon a formidable combination. When Simon claimed in his account of those years that if some action or other was contemplated 'My Lords always did me the honor of inviting my recommendations', it could be assumed as most probable that it was 'My Lords' who had taken their instructions from their Chief Medical Officer. This perhaps helps to explain why, seen through the eyes of public health administrators of later times who had been granted nothing like the same freedom of action, Simon's period of service at the Privy Council often appears as 'his golden age', with 'all the charm and brilliance of academic life'.

Among the obligations for which Simon expressed his indebtedness to the Vice-President was Lowe's having 'powerfully promoted the working of the department as against the unavoidable difficulties of its official novelty': a diplomatically coded reference to the hostility and non-cooperation he had to contend with in the early stages, not least because 'the functions which the Act of 1858 required the Privy Council to fulfil were supplementary in an essential sense to certain [others?] which the Poor Law Board was fulfilling'. The 'essential sense' was that the Poor Law Board still controlled the contracts made with medical practitioners for performing public vaccination, and was therefore well placed to frustrate measures intended by the Privy Council to introduce improvements in the service. Some delicate manoeuvring was called for which need not be described in detail; his own summary of 'the proceedings of the Lords in Council in respect of their share of the divided responsibility' will suffice:

First – they defined in technical *Instructions* what should in future be understood as a proper fulfilment of the contractor's undertaking to 'vaccinate' [...] they opened educational vaccinating-stations where medical students could receive the instruction, or be examined as to their competence. Second [...] they laid down the rules which ought to be observed in the appointment of times and places for public vaccination. Thirdly, with a view to the maintenance of the general supply of lymph, they arranged that the National Vaccine Establishment (which of late years had been tending to failure) should have [...] a sufficient number of carefully selected stations...[5]

The tendency to failure was not unconnected with the fact that since 1840 the Establishment had been under the aegis of the Poor Law Board, and in general Simon's terse summary fails to mention the sullen obstruction that his proposals had to contend with at the hands of the Board.

Simon acknowledged the extent to which, in bringing about these and other changes, he had profited 'by much special consultation' with experts in the field, notably Ceely, Marson and Seaton, the last named of whom became his closest collaborator for more than a decade and ultimately succeeded him briefly as Medical Officer. Seaton was an Englishman who like many of his contemporaries received his medical education in Scotland. After spending a few years in Kent as surgeon to the North Aylesford Union he joined a practice in London, where he remained for some twenty years. Having developed a great interest in the subject of epidemic disease, especially smallpox, he became, along with Simon and Marson among others, a founder of the Epidemiological Society and a member of its Council. As honorary secretary of the Society's committee on smallpox and vaccination he was largely responsible for drafting the report to Parliament that inspired the Vaccination Act of 1853. His *Vaccination Handbook*, published in 1868, achieved a status and authority similar to those of Simon's *Vaccination Papers*. The obituary notices marking his death in 1880 inevitably stressed his positive qualities: 'great power of organisation, rare tact and judgment combined with firmness [...] which enabled him to conciliate much of the opposition with which he would otherwise have had to contend' (*Lancet*). The *British Medical Journal*, assessing him as a good disciplinarian, paid tribute to 'his thorough honesty and his upright and sterling character', and gave him credit 'to a very great extent for the improvements in vaccination achieved in the preceding twenty years'. Acquaintance with his writings suggests a rather more tetchy side to him, somewhat bureaucratic, impatient and censorious; his favourite adjective, referring to shortcomings in the performance of vaccination, seems to have been 'scandalous'. It was widely accepted that some passages in documents published over Simon's name owed much of their abrasiveness to Seaton's pen.

His professional relationship with Simon began in an informal way during the last years of the General Board of Health and developed rapidly with the change of regime at the Privy Council. The Act that brought about the transfer empowered the Council to make 'inquiries in relation to any matters concerning the public health'. Inquiries need inquirers, and it was in this capacity that Simon found employment for his talented and enthusiastic colleague. The plan was for the medical department to 'enter upon a minute survey of public vaccination' in every district of England and Wales. Seaton was enlisted as a full-time inspector to launch the inquiry in London where smallpox, always endemic, had erupted once again into an epidemic. Since Parliament, while authorizing inquiries, had neglected, not for the first time, to provide money for what it had authorized, a reluctant Treasury had to be cajoled into approving a way of funding the exercise, according to which Seaton was paid on a daily basis at five guineas a day for what, it had been assumed by everyone except presumably Simon and Seaton, would be a short-term appointment. Once the door had been pushed ajar by this means Simon was able by degrees to force it open more widely, employing Seaton on a much more extended inquiry and eventually adding three more inspectors, all on a daily rate of three guineas, on a survey that lasted for five years from 1860 to 1864, and that provided both a comprehensive picture of the parlous state of public vaccination throughout the country and a merciless indictment of a sloppily conceived and incompetently executed piece of legislation, the Vaccination Act of 1853. The findings of the four inspectors, Seaton, Stevens, Sanderson and Buchanan, all of whom went on to hold high office in the public health service, were set out, supported by mountains of statistics, in Simon's annual reports to the Privy Council and attained the status of classics of their kind, constituting, one of the inspectors wrote, 'the first considerable compendium and thesaurus of social medicine in the language'.

In his recollections of those years Simon conceded that, although it had undertaken investigations into a great variety of topics, the medical department might appear to an outsider to have been 'bestowing disproportionate care on the one speciality of vaccination'.[6] There were, for example, diseases chiefly of childhood which at different times destroyed many more young lives annually than smallpox. Gale noted that in every hot summer for at least 300 years before 1911 'there was an enormous mortality among infants from diarrhoea [...]

In 1911 31,900 deaths among infants under one year were ascribed to diarrhoea and enteritis.' William Farr wrote in the Annual Report to the Registrar General for 1863 that 'the great reigning disease for the year' had been scarlatina (scarlet fever), which killed 30,475, mainly children. In the following year he recorded that 'whooping cough stands now next in fatality among children's diseases to scarlatina, and its mortality is never in any year low'. A table of 'Causes of Death' for each year from 1853 to 1862 showed that in 1858 the figures were: smallpox 6,460; whooping cough 11,648; scarlatina 30,317.

Simon's defence for the apparently low level of concern generated by these horrifying statistics was that 'the power of vaccination to prevent smallpox was already so familiarly known to the general public, that the knowledge seemed peculiarly to claim administrative recognition, in that one speciality preventive medicine had ripened to a point at which the legislature had become able to expressly apply it'. The state of the law as to compulsory vaccination 'had made it urgent, as a point of honour between government and people, that public vaccination in all parts of the country should be as good as the best knowledge and the utmost painstaking could render it'.

That was a retrospective assessment. The problem facing Simon in 1859 was that both the state of the law and the state of public vaccination had an immense distance to travel before achieving acceptance, still less approval, among the 'lower orders' for whose alleged benefit governments were legislating.

CHAPTER 11

THE PRESENT NON-SYSTEM

Some years after Simon's death a former colleague wrote of him that he never took part personally in any 'close epidemic inquiry', and failed to understand how much time and work was called for. This judgement was presumably based on personal observation, yet it is difficult to believe, studying the reports of the investigations carried out by his team of four vaccination inspectors, that he could have remained unaware of the labour involved in collecting the information.

One inspector's annual report showed that during the year under review his inquiries had extended over the counties of Cambridge, Derby, Huntingdon, Leicester, Northampton, Warwick and Nottingham. This territory included 93 unions, subdivided into 457 vaccination districts. He had conferred with 373 public vaccinators, 235 sub-district registrars, the majority of the ministers of religion and with 'many people of influence living in the different districts'. He had personally examined the conditions as to vaccination (i.e. the marks on the arms) of 46,871 children in national, parochial, workhouse and other schools, and of 'a great many in and about the dwellings of the poor and neglected', classifying them as 'good, indifferent or bad'. In another year the same inspector, Dr Stevens, was allotted as his sphere of operation the 79 unions in the West Riding of Yorkshire, Lancashire, Cheshire and part of Cumberland, 'embracing a population of 4,498,695, extending over 3,697,342 acres, divided into 507 vaccination districts [served by] 511 public vaccinators and 366 sub-district registrars'. In addition to the routine work of inspecting the quantity and quality of vaccination marks, if any, of all the children in this vast area,

I had interviews with the clerks to the guardians, several of the guardians and some magistrates in all the unions visited; and I have had conversations with 403 public vaccinators and 344 sub-registrars, as well as with clergymen and other persons having influence. In visits to schools I have carefully explained to the teachers [...] the nature of my inquiry and the appearances that should be found on the arms of the successfully vaccinated, and I have pointed out to them the groundlessness of the prejudices against vaccination.[1]

The other three inspectors showed similar assiduity, for which they received their three, or in Seaton's case five, guineas a day.

To those who had drafted the Vaccination Act of 1853 the procedure laid down must have appeared simplicity itself. The guardians in every union would divide it into districts and appoint in each one a convenient place for the performance of vaccination, giving notice of the times when the medical officer or practitioner – the public vaccinator or contractor – would be in attendance. When the birth of a child was registered the sub-registrar of the district would notify the parents of the requirement to have it vaccinated within three months. When the vaccination of the child could be shown – by inspection eight days later – to have been successful the contractor would hand a certificate to the parents and send a duplicate to the registrar, who would enter the details in the prescribed register.

The vaccination service therefore depended chiefly on three groups of persons: the guardians, who were elected by the ratepayers and under the control of the Poor Law Board were responsible for making the administrative arrangements; the contractors, who had a dual allegiance to the Poor Law Board for their conditions of service and to the Privy Council for the satisfactory performance of their medical function; and the sub-registrars, responsible to the Registrar General's department for the paper work on which the smooth running of the service depended. To these could be added the parents, whose compliance was necessary, and the magistrates, who would have to deal with defaulters and impose the penalties specified in the Act. This was the system, or as Seaton called it, no doubt in a fit of exasperation, 'the present non-system', which Simon was determined to improve or, if necessary, supersede after first demonstrating what a shambles it was.

One of the most obvious conclusions to be drawn from the exhaustive inspections was that the division of the country into vaccination districts and the issuing of contracts to public vaccinators had been undertaken in the most perfunctory manner, being based simply on the existing arrangements for administering the Poor Law. No allowance had been made for the differences between the two functions with the result that, as Simon stressed in his report for 1861, the contracts for vaccination were 'practically worthless'. In some districts the times and places appointed for the attendance of vaccinators were far too numerous, in others not numerous enough, in which event a shortage of vaccinifers (involuntary donors of lymph) could cause the arm-to-arm procedure to break down. In other unions the stipulation that vaccination stations should be 'conveniently situated' was ignored and parents were often required to travel long distances, usually on foot, to reach the appointed station in their own district when a station near their own home would have done just as well.

The monitoring of contracts was equally chaotic. Finding that what they had undertaken was either impractical or inconvenient, contractors took to making their own arrangements. Some dispensed with official vaccination stations altogether, going from place to place extemporizing a station at some convenient cottage or perhaps at a public house. Appointments made by vaccinators at their own residences were, in Seaton's curt phrase, 'mostly fictitious'. Sanderson commented on 'a general carelessness and complete absence of method... the contractor will make some such statement as "I catch them as I can", or "when I see an unvaccinated child I do it", and as regards inspection, "I look in next time I pass that way", or "if a vaccination doesn't take I hear about it".' There was no superior control, Simon concluded, and 'contracts have come to be regarded (except their stipulations for payment) as of no obligatory force'.

The chief sufferers from this muddle were of course the parents. They did not mind going long distances, Seaton remarked (offering no proof), but they did object to waiting and not seeing the vaccinator:

We had frequent evidence of children being taken to the public vaccinator at the appointed times and places without finding him or a legal substitute in his place; or when he was found there was no lymph for vaccination; or if there was lymph it was not of the kind that parents like, fresh from the arm of another child. (Seaton and Buchanan, London)[2]

I met with more than one instance in which parents have been summoned for non-vaccination of children, and magistrates, anxious to see the law upheld, have felt they could not justly inflict the penalty because it was proved that the appointments of the vaccinator had not been observed. (Seaton)[3]

As with the introduction of free vaccination in 1840 many guardians had saved their parishioners extra expense by appointing as their public vaccinator the existing parish medical officer, at a lower than usual rate of pay, 'the place and time of attendance for vaccination being usually identical with those fixed for attendance of pauper cases of sickness'.

What mattered as much as the quantity of vaccination was the quality. How well had the job been done? What constituted 'good' or 'successful' vaccination? This was a problem that Jenner had been aware of from the earliest days. 'The principle of vaccination is good,' he wrote in 1819, 'but its application has been bad, and continues to be so.' Much of the blame at that time lay with the amateur philanthropists who had seized upon his 'discovery' and practised it with unrestrained and uninstructed enthusiasm. For some years many of his own professional colleagues had little better understanding of what they were doing or how it should be done. He tried to stem the tide of incompetence, going, it was later argued, too far in the opposite direction, making the operation appear more difficult than it was as a way of protecting himself from his critics.

Attempts were made from time to time to educate would-be vaccinators in the basic technique of the arm-to-arm method but none of them went to the heart of the matter. A speaker at a conference of the Provincial Medical and Surgical Association in 1838 put the position plainly: 'I fear that at present we possess no permanent sign or an infallible proof of the full and protective action of vaccination having taken place in the system. The only sign that has hitherto been relied on is the scar which has been left upon the arm after the operation.' A year later the emphasis had shifted but only towards reliance on negative proof: 'though the presence of a perfect cicatrix is not a sure sign of protection its absence must be held to speak strongly against the existence of vaccine influence'.

There the matter seems to have rested until the imminent arrival of compulsion forced it back on to the agenda. When the Bill was brought forward in 1853 the *Lancet*, having listed some of the well-advertised problems, fastened on a fundamental one:

> no compulsory enactment can take effect with either justice or propriety, unless due provision be made for determining who is vaccinated and who is not. The insertion of lymph is one thing, vaccination inoculation another. The latter only is protective; the former may lead to protection in one case, in another it may prove inert, in a third injurious... The appointment of an inspector, therefore, approved by the Vaccine Board or some other competent medical authority, becomes a necessary provision, in order to carry out the object with certainty.[4]

In spite of this warning the Act as passed left the contractor as the best judge of his own success: no provision was made for an independent assessment of his handiwork.

The arrival on the scene of Simon and his quartet of inspectors did not contribute materially to a solution of the problem. In its absence attention was increasingly concentrated on the cicatrix and the development of an acceptable statistical correlation between the visible aftermath of the operation and the observed resistance of the vaccinee over a period of time to an attack of smallpox.

By 1859 when Seaton, the first of the inspectors, took to the road an unchallenged orthodoxy reigned. The *sine qua non* lay in the production of 'the true Jennerian vesicle' as described in the annual report for 1825 of the National Vaccine Establishment: 'it should be distinctly defined, perfectly spherical, indented, radiated and no larger than a common wafer. The diameter of the scar is less important than its circular and well-defined edge.' The minutest deviation from the perfect character of a vesicle (admired by Seaton for its 'beauty') meant, in Simon's view, that it was not to be relied on as a protection against smallpox.

The next question to be settled was 'how many?', that is to say how many punctures in the arm of the vaccinee, leading to how many clearly discernible scars? In Jenner's and Moore's day this was a matter of little importance: the assumption appears to have been that one properly carried out insertion of the lancet was sufficient; by mid-century a more closely defined dogma was taking over. Marson, one of the most highly respected authorities, set out in a document reproduced in Simon's *Vaccination Papers*, his 'mode of vaccinating': 'The arm to be operated on should be firmly grasped with the left hand of the operator [...] the lancet being already charged, the lymph should be introduced [...] in five punctures – the number I recommend – from half to three fourths of an inch apart.' A dozen or so years later Marson's recommendation had become, in Seaton's *Handbook*, a specific injunction. 'In vaccinating by puncture *not less than* five should be made, and they should be at a distance of half an inch from each other' [original italics]. Each puncture would, or should, result in a cicatrix with a normal area 'seldom short of a tenth of a square inch', leaving its indelible mark as evidence of vaccination properly performed and, except in rare cases, of immunity to smallpox assured.

Here, then, at least for Simon's inspectors, was the definitive solution to the problem: when is vaccination successful, and how do you know? 'Test the question in which way soever we may, the result is in favour of producing four vesicles at least [...] with lymph that leaves good permanent cicatrices.' That was the theory; the performance all too often fell short of the desire. 'Vaccination', Simon warned sternly, 'is not a mere easy trick of the fingers [...] precaution and minute care are necessary.' Marson supplied the harsh statistics:

> With good lymph and the observance of all proper precautions an expert vaccinator should not fail in his attempts to vaccinate above once in 150 times; yet a large number of those who take upon themselves the duty think they do well if they succeed, however imperfectly, five times out of six. Patients often present themselves with smallpox at the hospital, who state that they have been cut five, six, eight times or more. This is a great evil.[5]

Seaton told of a highly qualified medical practitioner who, according to his own account, 'could not make his vaccination succeed more than 4 times out of 5'. What the quality of private vaccination was like no one seemed either to know or care.

In the meantime inspectors had a benchmark against which to assess the state of the nation's arms, or at least those of its children, after nearly a decade of compulsory vaccination. Their annual reports justified the worst accusations of its critics:

> Not one tenth part of the vaccinated children had that all but complete protection which four proper scars have been found to give. (Seaton: Yorkshire)[6]

> In Dowlais, in the union of Merthyr Tydfil [...] the vaccination of children of 3 to 7 years of age was scandalously bad. Some [...] was nothing more than a sham. (Seaton)[7]

> Only 3% [of children] had four typical cicatrices, 6.8 had three equally good, 26.7 had two, 25.5 had one, 15 were quite unprotected; and the amount of [their] immunity from death was very slight. (Stevens: Derbyshire, Shropshire, Staffordshire)[8]

> In a village in Gloucestershire, where vaccination has long been performed by an unqualified assistant, almost all the children in the school exhibit unsightly oblong scars such as might have been produced by an instrument having a blunt jagged edge. In a neighbouring town [...] the scars were in general not only very small, but so far from typical that they could scarcely be recognised as vaccination scars at all. (Sanderson)[9]

At Lambourn the peculiarity of the scars was clearly attributable to the usual method of insertion practised, described by the contractor as consisting of making 'a prod into the integument'. (Sanderson)[10]

In one district where vaccination was particularly bad I found some of it had been performed by the female housekeeper of the late public vaccinator. (Seaton: Cornwall)[11]

In his long report to the Privy Council and the Local Government Board on the great world pandemic of smallpox of 1870–73, Seaton blamed its severity in England on the years of 'inefficient, almost useless vaccination' to which Marson had drawn attention. Not only had public vaccinators preferred the easy option of using dried or preserved lymph, which was notoriously less reliable than that provided by the more demanding arm-to-arm method; they had been 'still content with endeavours to produce sometimes one, frequently two, and at most three vaccination vesicles', instead of the recommended four.

Practitioners who had vaccinated in that way all their lives [...] 'couldn't see why' they should change their practice, nor 'why' one vesicle shouldn't be as good as a dozen: and others who were willing to make a change had their troubles sometimes in the prejudices of parents [...] who could not 'see why' the doctor should be introducing new-fangled ways.[12]

Forty years went by: the arm-to-arm method of vaccination was superseded, compulsion, although remaining a legal requirement, virtually ceased to exist, and smallpox in Britain became an increasingly rare disease. In 1911 the leading authority, Copeman, contributing an article on 'Vaccination' to the 11th edition of the *Encyclopaedia Britannica*, admitted that

it is somewhat unfortunate that there exists no official definition of what constitutes 'successful vaccination', and in consequence it is open to any practitioner to give a certificate of successful vaccination where but one minute vesicle may have been produced. It is to be feared that such certificates are too frequently given, and it cannot be too strongly urged that vaccination of this sort involves incomplete protection.[13]

In their intensive investigations Simon's inspectors consulted guardians, contractors, registrars, clergymen, magistrates and teachers; the one part of the population whose opinions they did not deliberately seek were the parents of the children whose arms they were subjecting to such close scrutiny, but it did not follow that they learned nothing of interest from that source. As Seaton admitted, many parents had firm opinions and didn't hesitate to express them.

His own conclusion was that among parents there was little open hostility to vaccination, but rather 'indifference and a desire to procrastinate'. Neglect was to be put down to idleness, and the notion that 'so long as smallpox was not present there was no real necessity for vaccination, which interfered with the parents' occupation and made the children poorly [...] If they consented earlier it was out of kindness to the doctor.' Stevens detected apathy but also a tendency on the part of parents to believe that they were conferring a privilege on the vaccinator by allowing him to vaccinate their children, and expected something in return – 'a bottle of medicine, etc.' Buchanan came across 'a widely spread notion that the vaccinator got some advantage from their children and that they were entitled to some part of it'; they were 'minded that he should at least have a bit of trouble for his money, so they made him repeat his visit two or three times, till at last perhaps he got tired of it'.

The great hindrance to getting the job done properly came from parents who tried, often successfully, to dictate to the vaccinator how many punctures should be made in their child's arm. The common preference was for only one, which he would settle for rather than risk the child remaining completely unprotected. Another form of obstruction, not so serious in the long run, was caused by parents objecting to the vaccinator's choice of vaccinifer, and demanding that he select a child whom they knew and whose health they could feel confidence in.

In the prevailing state of vaccination parents may well have seen the whole thing as little more than a game in which their wits were pitted against those of the authorities, or at least the vaccinator. Legal proceedings, Seaton asserted, were seldom called for 'when parents are made thoroughly to understand that [...] "the law is not to be trifled with"'. Sanderson, who emerges as a more shrewd and sympathetic observer, reported successful prosecutions in several districts, but was unsure about their long-term advantage:

The expedient of frightening parents into compliance, even if at first it should appear efficacious, is apt soon to fall into contempt. The other plan of soliciting or 'touting' for vaccination cases is so unworthy and derogatory that even if success could be obtained by it, it would be too dearly purchased.

Sanderson's veiled caution against too much reliance on heavy-handed tactics is unlikely, coming from such a source, to have gone down well at the top level; as time went by it was increasingly disregarded, with consequences that were unfortunate and far-reaching.

Much of the blame for non-compliance with the Act can be laid at the door of its framers. Well-heeled themselves, living lives largely insulated from the concerns of the mass of the population, they can have had little understanding of the daily struggles and problems of the 'lower orders' who were the objects of their good intentions; that inter-ference, mentioned by Seaton, with the parents' occupation, when the pressure of earning a living meant that attendance at a vaccination station not once but twice in eight days could be a costly distraction. Sanderson, for example, tactfully drew attention to the importance of choosing times for vaccination 'which will interfere as little as possible with the agricultural interests of the district'. There were, according to one investigation, '1,000,000 persons in this country who are engaged in a daily struggle with pauperism', with the looming presence of a well-run workhouse to spur them on to greater efforts. It is not difficult to imagine the state of mind of a farm labourer trying to get by on twelve shillings a week, supplemented by the pence brought in by a wife and six or seven children, and threatened with a fine amounting to well over a week's wages for not having the latest arrival vaccinated – however shoddily.

There was one cause that everyone, not least Simon, recognized as having destroyed whatever effectiveness the compulsory Vaccination Act might have had: 'Owing to the utter and universal failure of the intended register of vaccination the failure of the other parts of the system cannot be accurately measured.' The registrars were not to blame: they usually performed their functions 'with great assiduity', Buchanan recorded. Stevens saw them as 'a very intelligent body anxiously desirous of doing their duty, and for the most part doing it very regularly'. The roots of the disaster went much more deeply.

The problem lay in the excessive amount of clerical work demanded of the contractor, who had not only to keep a record of every vaccina-tion he performed but, following every inspection, to fill in two certificates, one for the parents and the other for the registrar to enter in his record book. In practice the certificates were either not written or not sent, with the result that many pages of the registrar's book remained blank, he didn't receive the fees due to him and the whole purpose of the procedure was defeated.

Among the most trenchant critics of the system was William Farr. In 1867, with a new Bill in the offing, he delivered a speech to a branch meeting of the British Medical Association that included a scathing attack on the Act of 1853 and those responsible for it:

> Nothing can be conceived more impractical [than its registration clauses]. Anyone who had the slightest administrative capacity could have foretold its failure [...] What hindrance these certificates throw in the way of a man whose [vaccination] station is full of children, or who wants to get away to other patients or to a woman at a distance in labour, we can easily conceive.[14]

Farr was quite clear where the blame lay for this farcical situation. The Act was 'a piece of amateur legislation for which as far as I know no government department is responsible'. The Bill had been introduced in the Lords, and the minister nominally in charge of its passage through the Commons was Palmerston, the Home Secretary. The Registrar General had convinced him, according to Farr, that the registration clauses 'would not work', and he had intended to propose that they should be dropped in committee, but happened unfortunately to be absent from the morning sitting at the end of the session, with the result that the Bill had been passed as it stood, epitomizing the indifference and incompetence with which Jenner's 'great discovery' was habitually dealt with by the legislature.

There were other problems that frustrated the attempts of registrars to carry out their duties, one of the chief being the inadequacy of the Act that had called their own profession into existence. The first step in the vaccination procedure was, or should have been, the registration of the birth of the child, but the Act of 1836 'for registering the Births, Deaths and Marriages in England', unlike its counterparts in Scotland and Ireland, was extraordinarily ambiguous on the subject of births. Clause 19 provided that 'the parent or occupier of any house or tenement in England in which a birth [...] shall happen *may* within forty-two days next after the day of birth [...] give notice of such birth to the registrar of the district' (author's italics). Clause 20 required the parent or occupier within forty-two days of the birth to 'give information, upon being requested to do so by the registrar [...] of the several particulars required to be known touching the birth'. The penalty for failing to complete the necessary formalities within the stipulated time limit was a fine of fifty pounds: except that a solemn declaration made within six months of the due date would be 'lawful' and presumably allow exemption from the penalty.

Early reports by the Registrar General gave warning of the consequences of the loose wording of the Act, which in effect threw upon district registrars the responsibility for securing the registration of a birth:

> At present [1844] I am well aware that many thousands of births
> annually escape registration: increased exertions on the part of
> registrars may effect much; but in my opinion *all* [original italics]
> the births will not be registered until by law it be made compulsory
> to give notice [...] of a birth having occurred.[15]

The annual report for the following year drew attention yet again to
the anomaly but despite the appointment of four inspectors to pay
regular visits to every district in England, predictions that the situation
would improve were shown to be hopelessly optimistic. Another thirty
years had to pass before an Act, inspired by the need to deal with the
scandal of baby-farming, rectified the inexplicable omission.

In the meantime sub-registrars had to cope as best they could with
the problem of locating every infant born in their district. Having registered their existence the harassed official had then to keep track of
them for vaccination purposes. Between the birth of the child and the
date by which it should have been vaccinated the family might well
have moved away, leaving no address at which they might be found.
Mobility among the labouring classes in the latter part of the century
was a more common fact of life than the framers of legislation appear
to have allowed for, and not all of the migrants and immigrants were
'tramps', in the derogatory sense of the term. The pseudonymous
'Journeyman Engineer' (Thomas Wright) in his classic work, *The Great
Unwashed*, tried to put the record straight. The word 'tramp', as understood among the working classes, he explained, meant simply 'a
working man "on the road" in search of work'. Lacking the means of
paying for railway or other means of conveyance he would simply set
off on his own two feet, joining the great fraternity of travellers of
whom Wright himself had at least twice formed part.

> All kinds of workmen are occasionally obliged to 'take to the road',
> but the class who are most frequently found on the tramp are the
> mechanics who are members of trade unions [...] Even under the
> most advantageous circumstances going on the road is anything
> but pleasant, and is regarded as a mode of looking for work only to
> be adopted as a last resource.[16]

The importance of these men as far as registrars were concerned lay
not in the possibility of their carrying smallpox around the country,
which they were often accused of, but in their influence on the vacci-

nation system and its chaotic statistics: the father 'on the road', the mother keeping the home and a newborn baby in good order with practically no resources, but with a printed form that in all probability she couldn't read, though she knew it threatened her absent spouse, in theory, with a fine impossible to pay if they unwittingly fell foul of the law in some way.

In practice the provisions made for the punishment of defaulters were in the same state of chaos as much of the rest of the Act. Lowe had largely undermined them by dropping from the 1859 Act the clause that would have allowed proceedings to be taken on the complaint of registrars, public vaccinators or officers, the cost to be defrayed out of the union funds. His attempt to restore the situation in 1861, with an Act empowering guardians to appoint 'some person' to institute and conduct proceedings, failed because it was wholly permissive and left guardians to decide whether or not to prosecute, in the knowledge that if they did they were still likely to have to bear the cost. Stevens was told by the clerk to the guardians in Halifax that 'no proceedings had been taken, and he assured me that none would be attempted because there was no possibility of proving the service upon the parent of the notice required [...] inasmuch as no copy was retained'. In Liverpool, where proceedings had been taken on several occasions, 'the magistrates took every conceivable objection and quashed them if possible [...] registrars had great difficulty in proving that the person to whom the notice was given was the parent, or that the person summoned was really the person who had received the notice'. In several unions the mother received the notice while the father was away at some distance at work on a railway line or in a mine: the magistrates would not convict because the father would be liable to pay a fine and might be assumed to be ignorant of his liability.

A great deal depended on the attitude of magistrates. In one union in Surrey 'the magistrates had expressed their determination to inflict another penalty to the full amount in case of continued opposition'; in neighbouring Hampshire 'the magistrates declined to grant a summons on the ground that the offenders were too poor to pay a fine'. In Derbyshire a contractor had taken it upon himself to instigate proceedings, as allowed by the Act, 'but from ignorance of details was unsuccessful and had to pay the costs'. In Cambridge a registrar took proceedings against a person who then complied with the law: 'the registrar was not paid his costs, but a demand was made upon him as unsuccessful prosecutor to pay all the charges'.

There was almost universal dissatisfaction. Guardians had no right of access to the register of successful vaccinations to discover who was or was not vaccinated; the registers were wholly misleading anyway. A feeling existed among some guardians against prosecution 'as calculated to excite local prejudice and ill-will, and hinder rather than promote vaccination'; contractors, even when they tried to abide by the rules, were obstructed by aggressive parents, and felt that vaccination had become 'the most detested part of their work'; registrars complained that since the Act of 1853 had placed so many extra duties upon them for such inadequate payment 'their office was hardly worth holding'. Even Simon's inspectors, for all their official status, were impotent when it came to a head-on collision with uncooperative guardians, who could always appeal to the Poor Law Board. In Hull, Seaton pointed out to the guardians 'the inconvenience and disadvantages of their existing arrangements' and suggested improvements. 'I was subsequently informed by letter from the clerk that "the guardians appointed a sub-committee to consider the whole question", and the committee, after several meetings, were unable to "recommend to the board any improvements" [...] and that no alteration had been made'.[17]

CHAPTER 12

TOTIES QUOTIES

Simon's assessment of the four-year campaign of inspection was that it provided 'an account of the working of our present vaccination laws which [...] offers such a basis as there has never yet been for effective legislation against small-pox'. Stevens, speaking for those who, like himself, had been doing the arduous leg-work, took the less complacent view that it was entirely hopeless to attempt to secure to the people 'such an amount of protection as they have the right to claim [...] from the law as at present administered'. The cause lay with no one person or with any one union – it was simply 'the system' that was at fault. 'Gentlemen of influence' in every district had without exception expressed to him their opinion that 'no improvement could possibly be effected under the existing Vaccination Acts'. There could be no disagreement, except perhaps from the anti-vaccination lobby which had shown its head above the parapet a few years earlier, but had still to get itself organized; the mass of parents, unconsulted as usual, continued to treat the whole issue with the 'indifference and idleness' of which Seaton had recently accused them.

In February 1866 a Bill to 'consolidate and amend the statutes relating to vaccination in England' was brought forward, sent to a select committee and returned in a revised form in June. In normal circumstances the Act would probably have been on the statute book by the end of the year; but the circumstances, once again, though not abnormal, were unfavourable: a change of government caused it to be lost, but only temporarily. The incoming government, although not viewing it with much enthusiasm, revived it in 1867, a development that had a profound bearing on the history of compulsory vaccination. To understand why, a few steps must be retraced.

In 1864 the partnership of Simon and Lowe was dissolved for practical purposes following Lowe's departure from the administration. His only formal contribution to vaccination in the immediately preceding years was the passing of the Act of 1861, with which the lost clause of its predecessor of 1859 was retrieved. The effect was minimal. As Simon recognized in his report of 1861, 'a first touch of legal proceedings' was enough to conquer the parental inertia that accounted for so large a part of the infant population being left unvaccinated, but 'owing to the construction of the law that touch is in most cases absent. For how are legal proceedings to be paid for?' The Act was 'entirely permissive', and boards of guardians were unwilling to embark on prosecutions that might leave the ratepayers out of pocket.

At about this period Lowe made his mark in his major sphere of responsibility, education, with the only innovation for which, if at all, he is remembered today. At the time of his appointment as Vice-President a royal commission, chaired by Lord Newcastle, was considering how to improve the quality of education of the poorer classes. There was no question of making school attendances compulsory, only of raising the standard of teaching in schools receiving the government grant, by what a later age would recognize as the basis, at least, of a core curriculum – reading, writing and arithmetic. In a phrase that offered a close parallel to what was in progress elsewhere, the commissioners called for the launch of 'a searching examination by competent authority of every child in every school in the country' to see how well he or she was acquiring 'these indispensable elements of knowledge', and, in an ominous phrase, 'to make the prospects and position of the teacher dependent to a considerable extent on the results of this examination'. So was born the concept of 'payment by results', or, with the addition of a couple of redundant syllables, 'performance-related pay', which, in the face of bitter criticism and opposition from many in Parliament and the profession, was finally imposed in 1862.

Four years later a version of the same procedure was inaugurated in the second of the Vice-President's fiefdoms, vaccination. By this time Lowe had vacated the office, and there is some confusion as to who proposed the measure. Lowe himself, addressing the electors of the University of London in 1874, was in no doubt – 'I might take credit to myself for it' – and Simon's recollection was that 'the contrivance – a parliamentary grant for payment for results was founded on the hint of Mr Lowe's Education Code'. Lambert, ever eager to talk up Simon's achievements, agrees that 'Lowe claimed credit for the device', but seems to transfer it to Simon who 'hit on a characteristic mid-Victorian device' and 'primed' the chairman of a select committee that was considering proposals for a new Vaccination Act to incorporate it in its report.

The payments distributed by the Privy Council were intended, without placing an additional burden on the rates, to reward 'meritorious public vaccinators' with gratuities in excess of their contract receipts. The system came into force in 1867 with the distribution of £1,824. The largest payment to one vaccinator was £67.7s. 4d., and the smallest 15s. 4d. By 1875 the total had risen to £15,676. There was a noticeable difference between payment *by* results for teachers and payment *for* results for vaccinators. For the teacher, if the results were good, payment could rise or at least remain constant; if they were bad it could go down as an incentive to the recipient to do better. For medical practitioners good results could be rewarded: the bad vaccinator incurred no penalty, financial or otherwise.

Payment by, or for, results, though proposed in 1866, was not inaugurated until the following year as a small part of a piece of far-reaching legislation. Almost from the moment when vaccination of newborn infants was made compulsory a fundamental flaw in the concept had become apparent. A fine for default punished the parent but left the child unvaccinated and by implication unprotected from smallpox. No strategy for enforcing the law more strictly as it stood removed the obstacle. Lowe's Act of 1861 was, as Simon had recognized, a failure. Proposals by some militant boards of guardians to apply pressure by repeated prosecutions on the principle that the Act allowed proceedings to be 'taken at any time during which the parent is at fault' were countered by doubts in more cautious quarters as to the legality of prosecuting an offender more than once for the same offence.

The issue was put to the test in January 1864. William Stafford, a shoemaker living in Margate, had in the previous year been fined 2s. 6d., with 9s. costs, for failing to have his child vaccinated and had still not complied with the law. The local sub-registrar, Charles Pilcher, now launched a second prosecution in respect of the same child, submitting that the words 'at any time' must be construed to mean that a parent could be convicted again and again until he obeyed the law; in support of which contention Pilcher produced a statement from the vaccination department of the Privy Council. Stafford countered with the claim that he had paid one penalty and could not be prosecuted a second time. The justices upheld his argument on the ground that the principle that 'no man should be punished twice for the same offence must prevail in the absence of any express legislative enactment to the contrary'.[1]

The exact interpretation of the phase 'at any time' was disputed. Pilcher maintained that the words meant precisely what they said and had been introduced into the Act for the specific purpose of overriding the principle enshrined in an earlier statute, generally known as

'Jarvis's Act', that provided that no prosecution could be undertaken more than six months after the offence complained of had been committed. The justices took the view that the words in question must be construed strictly in accordance with Jarvis, which could not be set aside; they therefore found for Stafford, but agreed that the case should go to appeal, where Lord Chief Justice Cockburn upheld their decision. The continuous neglect of a child's vaccination was a mischief, but if the child was not vaccinated within the period prescribed 'the offence is complete'. There was no provision for a second notice by the registrar, and it did not meet the case of a continuation of neglect: 'This can only be remedied by fresh legislation.'

Pilcher v. Stafford presented the vaccination department with a challenge that it was only too ready to accept. Some indication of the steps proposed was given in April 1866 during the committee stage of the Bill referred to above, which had been introduced in February by Lowe's successor as Vice-President, H. A. Bruce. Although there appeared to be an apprehension that some new principle was involved in it, that, Bruce assured the Commons, was an illusion. There were, however, minor improvements contemplated. For example, when a penalty had once been imposed, however trifling, the guardians hitherto could not prosecute for continued neglect; it was now proposed to give them the power to take further proceedings – a clear warning, if one were needed, that the Lord Chief Justice's hint had not fallen on deaf ears. In principle, Bruce explained, the Bill would make every man responsible for the non-vaccination of his own child, and as every child born since 1853 and not vaccinated remained unvaccinated in defiance of the law, there would be no hardship in enforcing the law against all parents who had disregarded it in the case of all children not above thirteen years of age.

A clause covering the question of repeated prosecutions had been incorporated in the Bill. The committee to which it was despatched took no evidence; the government, Bruce indicated firmly, would not agree to any tampering with the principle of the Bill. Its reappearance, heavily amended in detail, in the Commons on 1 June was followed almost immediately by the resignation of the Whig administration of Earl Russell and his replacement by the Tory Earl of Derby. In these circumstances the Bill was withdrawn, and not heard of officially until the following year when news of its imminent resurrection drew from anti-vaccinationists a memorial addressed to the Duke of Buckingham, the Lord President of the Council, in which they set out their objections in general to the practice of vaccination, referred specifically to the Bill with its threat of cumulative penalties 'and several other oppressive provisions', and drew attention to petitions presented to Parliament from time to time by parents alleging deaths of children from vaccination. The memorial was ordered by the House to be printed but had no effect on the progress of the Bill, which had already begun the final stage of its progress in the hands, this time, of the latest Vice-President for Education, Lord Robert Montagu, who was at pains to stress that it was 'in almost the words in which it had come down from the [previous year's] select committee'. Somewhat surprisingly, in view of the almost unanimous condemnation of the existing state of affairs by Simon's inspectors, Montagu asserted that 'the energy of the public vaccinators and of the local authorities' had supplied the defects of the Act of 1853 and 'made it a perfect Vaccination Act'[2] – in which case, it might have been asked, why was a new one needed? There were now four inspectors – Simon's quartet upgraded by some sleight of hand to full-time salaried civil servants – whose duty was to travel once every two years around the districts allotted to them. A clause proposed by Lowe made the system of paying for results a permanent one. The long-standing division of responsibility for vaccination between the Privy Council and the Poor Law Board was once again confirmed. Beyond this, apart from a bewildering manipulation of a mass of statistics that enabled him to assert with confidence that the measure would make it absolutely certain that 7,000 children would be saved from death by smallpox in a year, Montagu rested his case, conveying the impression that, in spite, no doubt, of intensive coaching by the staff of his medical council, he had not succeeded in wholly mastering his brief. His predecessor, Bruce, who had done the real spadework on the Bill, bore the brunt of the not very demanding attack now made on it. The only surprising feature of his performance was a passage on the subject of re-vaccination that led him to affirm that 'experience has shown that, as a general rule, vaccination once in a life-time was a sufficient safe-guard against small-pox'.

So the Bill completed its passage, became an Act, and took its place on the statute book on 12 August 1867 as 'An Act to consolidate and amend the laws relating to vaccination', with little apparent recognition among its sponsors of the potential for disruption now firmly embedded in it, in what Lambert described in words already quoted as its 'astounding' Clause 31, 'a savage cat-and-mouse provision totally unprecedented in health legislation'. This, filleted of as much as possible of its legal verbiage, is the gist of the 'infamous' clause:

If any registrar or any officer appointed by the guardians [...] shall give information in writing to a justice of the peace that he has reason to believe that any child under the age of fourteen years within the union [...] has not been successfully vaccinated, and that he has given notice to the parent [...] to procure its being vaccinated, and that this notice has been disregarded, the justice may summon such parent to appear with the child before him [...] and upon the appearance, if the justice shall find, after such examination as he may deem necessary, that the child has not been vaccinated, nor has already had the small-pox, he may, if he sees fit, make an order [...] directing such child to be vaccinated within a certain time; and if at the expiration of such time the child shall not have been so vaccinated, or shall not be shown to be then unfit to be vaccinated, or to be insusceptible of vaccination, the person upon whom such order shall have been made shall be proceeded against summarily, and, unless he can show some reasonable ground for his omission to carry the order into effect, shall be liable to a penalty not exceeding twenty shillings.

Lambert asserts that even Simon 'had qualms' about the justice and necessity of the clause, which bears all the hallmarks of Seaton's handiwork. In the section of his *Handbook of Vaccination*, published in 1868, which deals with the duties of various officials under the act, Seaton appears in his true colours as a disciplinarian:

What immediate steps should be taken in cases of default of one kind or the other [...] will depend on the instructions which each Board of Guardians may give to its officer. But it would be an utter subversion of the declared object of the law to allow any person to escape unpunished who continued to neglect its requirements. The words of the Act are positive that Guardians *shall cause proceedings to be taken* against the persons in default [Seaton's italics].[3]

Guardians might in the first instance issue warnings to the parents, '[b]ut if there be any neglect of such warning, proceedings ought then by no means to be delayed: and in districts in which anything like habitual neglect exists, my experience satisfies me that public examples will be indispensable.'

There was an immediate outcry against the Act by anti-vaccinationists, who began to form organizations to coordinate opposition to it, but the full implications of Clause 31 were not confirmed until the following year, when it was invoked amid widespread publicity to entrap the Revd H. T. Allen, an impoverished Primitive Methodist minister from St Neots in Huntingdonshire. Allen had five children and on conscientious grounds had refused to have them vaccinated. According to his own account he had been committed to prison, but on paying a fine of £5.20s for each child, was released. In May 1869 the sub-registrar of the district, known to posterity only as Worthy, laid an information before the justices of the peace that Allen had disobeyed an order to have his daughter, Eliza, vaccinated, she being under the age of thirteen at the time.[4]

The court heard that Allen had already been fined two months previously for disobeying a similar order in respect of Eliza. His defence was that, in accordance with the judgement delivered by Lord Chief Justice Cockburn in *Pilcher v. Stafford*, he could not be convicted again for the same offence. The justices this time decided that the previous conviction had no bearing on the present charge, which formed a separate offence covered by Clause 31 of the Act, which appeared to them to have been inserted with the object of preventing the unsatisfactory situation found to exist when *Picher v. Stafford* was decided. A second line of defence was also dismissed. A medical practitioner, Dr W. J. Collins, a prominent anti-vaccinationist, had issued a certificate in April 1869 stating that in his opinion Eliza was unfit for vaccination, but the certificate was for a limited period and no longer valid. Allen was found guilty and fined 7 shillings with costs. The case went to the court of appeal, where it was heard by the same Lord Chief Justice who had dealt with *Pilcher v. Stafford*.

The importance attached to the case by the government was indicated by the presence of the Solicitor General, who explained for the benefit of the court the difference between the wording and intentions of the relevant clauses of the Act. Under section 16 the parent was required to have his child vaccinated within three months; under section 29, if he had failed to do so, or failed without sufficient excuse to take the child back eight days after vaccination to have it examined, he was guilty of an offence and could suffer a penalty. There could be only one offence and one penalty. These provisions had been carried over into the present Act from the Act of 1853, and if Allen were being charged for offences under sections 16 and 29, *Pilcher v. Stafford* would be 'a case in point'; but, the Solicitor General explained, 'section 31 creates an offence of a different character'. In that section the period in which the child was to be vaccinated was not limited to three months, but extended up to fourteen years, and as the object of the legislation was to enforce vaccination fresh orders could be made and fresh penalties imposed so long as the parent continued to neglect to have the child vaccinated: 'He is not convicted for the same offence, but for a fresh and separate offence of not obeying an order to vaccinate.' Each order disobeyed, therefore, constituted a new and separate offence and could become the subject of a fresh conviction and penalty. The offender could be prosecuted, as the legal Latin phrase had it, *toties quoties*, meaning 'as many times as' he committed the offence.

Giving judgement the Lord Chief Justice could only go over the same ground again at greater length. He had at first been disposed to accept the argument that the powers given by section 31 could not be exercised *toties quoties*, but the Solicitor General had caused him to change his mind. 'The language [of the section] is general. I do not see anything to control it, and when we look to the intention of the legislature, I think we are bound to give a reasonable construction to this, which is evidently intended as a remedial Act'. He therefore held that the powers given by section 31 were not confined to one order or one conviction but that 'the proceedings may be repeated *toties quoties* so long as disobedience continues.'

CHAPTER 13

CROTCHETY PEOPLE

Allen v. Worthy opened the floodgates. Parents objecting to the vaccination of their children found themselves in court time and time again, paying fines and costs that for many of them amounted to a severe financial burden. Refusal or inability to pay could result in their possessions being seized or sold off, or even a prison sentence. Typical of those who faced what was for them a desperate moral dilemma was a parent who ascribed his eldest child's death to vaccination, no doubt without justification, and felt he must resist the compulsory vaccination of a second child. He was summoned, convicted and paid the full penalty, only to be forced through the same train of events a second time. 'What am I to do? I am a young man and cannot afford to pay 34 shillings every two or three months. I must either stifle my parental convictions and have my child poisoned or be ruined by continuing to refuse. They have threatened me again'.[1] As an opponent of the compulsory legislation remarked, what it accomplished in practice was that a parent might be 'imprisoned for ever'.

Shortly after the Act of 1867 was passed, but before *Allen v. Worthy* had revealed its full implications, the office of Vice-President for Education had changed hands again. Lord Derby had been supplanted as Prime Minister by Disraeli, and Disraeli, in December 1868, by Gladstone, for whom the pros and cons of compulsory vaccination were among the least of his preoccupations. The new Vice-President was W. E. Forster, the Quaker MP for Bradford, who by August 1870 was emerging from his long-drawn-out battle to secure the passage of his eponymous Education Act. As this struggle was reaching its climax a Bill was introduced by the anti-vaccinationist MP for Sunderland, John Candlish, which proposed that 'no more than two orders shall be made, under the thirty-first section of the Vaccination Act of 1867, for the vaccination of any one child', and also attempted to remove some confusion over certificates of unfitness for vaccination. The Bill made no progress but in response to the rising tide of anger and condemnation of the 'cat-and-mouse Act', accentuated by the ravages of the great smallpox pandemic that had broken out some months previously and was now at its height, the Home Secretary, and former Vice-President, H. A. Bruce, announced that in 1871 a select committee of the Commons would be set up 'to enquire into the operation of the [Vaccination] Act and report whether the said Act should be amended'. The chairman, wearing his vaccination hat, would be Forster, with, as his deputy, J. T. Hibbert, the member for Oldham and secretary to the Poor Law Board, an arrangement reflecting the divided control of the vaccination system that, in spite of continued opposition, had recently been confirmed yet again.

Among the other thirteen members of the committee the anti-vaccinationist cause was represented by some stalwart campaigners, including John Candlish, who had sat on the committee that considered the Bill of 1867; P. A. Taylor, representing Leicester, one of the most staunchly anti-vaccinationist cities in the country; and Jacob Bright, the member for Manchester, brother of the better known John and husband of Ursula, herself a vigorous critic of the Vaccination Act which, in common with most of its enemies, she stigmatized as 'a piece of class legislation'.[2] Their opponents were a more run-of-the-mill collection, with the possible exception of Montagu, the recent Vice-President, and the formidable figure of Dr (later Lord) Lyon Playfair, the member for Edinburgh and St Andrews Universities, one of the *éminences grises* of mid- and late Victorian Britain, whose most powerful intervention in the vaccination struggle was reserved for a later occasion.

The committee, for all its shortcomings, represented the first serious attempt to examine both the practical operation and the moral implications of the law on compulsory vaccination. It held fifteen sessions of which the first eight were devoted to hearing evidence from prominent anti-vaccinationists and no less than four of the remainder to an interrogation, by no means friendly at times, of John Simon. Ascribing the committee's existence to pressure from Forster, who is said to have shared his views on vaccination, Simon explained a decade or so later that its purpose was 'to afford to the anti-vaccinationists the full public hearing, long ago promised them, for all they could urge against vaccination and the vaccination law'. There were apparently suggestions that the committee had been 'rigged', presumably to show the opponents of vaccination in a bad light, but it was certainly true that this was the first occasion since the introduction of compulsion when leading members of the two camps had faced each other in person and in public, rather than in the constricting formality of what was often no more than a parliamentary charade.

Bearing in mind that a full transcript of the proceedings was printed, it is unfortunate that such subsequent references to it as are available are for the most part perfunctory, not to say one-sided. The anti-vaccinationists did not, as a group, do themselves justice, but with one or two exceptions were not the half-wits that selective quotation from their contribution makes them appear. One, a Quaker, who might have expected the Quaker chairman to follow his line of reasoning, suggested that conscientious objectors to compulsory vaccination might be allowed the option, granted to Quakers in matters of religion, to 'make an oath' or 'a simple declaration' to that effect, which would allow the legal obligation to be waived, freeing the objector from further harassment. This solution was in fact adopted a generation later by the Royal Commission on Vaccination as the only way round the fundamental impasse.

The same witness, Garth Wilkinson, something of a scholar and a widely respected practitioner of homoeopathy, seized the opportunity to denounce the undisguised class bias of the Vaccination Act. Was it not a fact, he was asked, that people in 'bad neighbourhoods' suffered immensely and died in large numbers if they were not vaccinated? Of course, he replied, but that wasn't peculiar to smallpox – they also suffered immensely from cholera, or from any epidemic disease: 'I attribute the fact that the unvaccinated die more (if they do so) and have small-pox very severely, to the fact that the unvaccinated are the poor, the wretched, the needy, the unclothed, the vicious.'[3] The chairman intervened: Why did he consider that the Vaccination Act, if carried out in its entirety, was more severe against the poorer classes than against the richer class? Because, as one honourable member said,

> when the purse is not there, the gaol is. If I were called upon to have a child vaccinated now I could to a certain extent pay fines once a fortnight, but a poor man cannot pay fines at all, and there-fore has to go to gaol at once. The law is quite unequal in what it does.

This was indisputable. At least one Member of Parliament had allegedly refused to have his children vaccinated and avoided falling foul of either section 29 or section 31.

Another witness, the Revd Hume-Rothery, not one of the more highly regarded opponents of compulsory vaccination, came up against a questioner less astute than himself and was able to put a universally

shared point of view: 'If the majority [of the population] believe vaccination to be a prophylactic they can protect themselves by practising
vaccination, and leave the minority to their own risks.' But if the
health of the majority were endangered by the minority being left to
themselves, would he still hold that opinion? 'If the majority, who say
vaccination is protective against disease, admit that they would be
endangered by the unvaccinated minority they concede the ground
which is claimed by the anti-vaccinationists; that vaccination is
useless.'[4] This, though undoubtedly true as far as it went, was unfortunately no answer to Simon's charge of 'omissional infanticide', the
infant in question having by definition no say in the matter.

The most effective critic of the law was, paradoxically, John
Candlish, who at the start of the proceedings vacated his seat on one
side of the table to appear as a witness on the other, supplying the
committee with evidence that had reached him concerning savage
treatment meted out to 'contumacious' parents. It was Candlish who,
as will become apparent, forced his parliamentary colleagues on the
pro-vaccination side to face up to the inherent inconsistency of their
position, when it came to the writing of their report.

Witnesses in support of the law as it stood included most of its
prominent begetters, chiefly Marson, Seaton and Simon. Their
evidence was limited in general to factual descriptions for the benefit of
lay members of the committee of its history, *raison d'être*, modus
operandi and unquestionable indispensability. Only one witness, D. P.
Fry, head of the legal department of the Poor Law Board for many
years, spoke with a degree of independence, supplying the occasional
much-needed corrective to the categorical assurances of the medical
staff of the Privy Council.

In one extraordinary episode Marson was only mildly reproved for
passing on as fact an allegation that, when mentioned by John Birch,
an opponent of Jenner, seventy years earlier as no more than an
opinion he had heard expressed had earned him bitter denunciation.
Marson was presumably aware, he was asked, that there was a strong
feeling and a great objection on the part of a number of people against
vaccination? 'Yes, I know there is, but I nearly always find that it is the
father who objects and not the mother, which makes it very suspicious
[...] The father would like the family as small as possible that he has to
work for. I'm afraid there's the bottom of it.'[5]

A noted physician, Sir William Jenner (no relation), assured the
committee that he had never seen any evil arising from vaccination,
except 'the local trouble. It may sometimes cause inflammation of the
arm, but nothing that the patient does not recover from in a week or

two.' Would he recommend every parent to have his child vaccinated early in life? 'I should think myself wicked and really guilty of a crime if I did not so recommend.'[6]

These experts were playing little more than walk-on parts in comparison with the virtuoso performance put on by John Simon, though this is passed over in one modern account with the brief comment that he 'gave his support to the act of 1867'; hardly surprising since the parts chiefly objected to were largely his creation. He was reported to have been 'exasperated' by the committee because of the extra burden of work it imposed upon him when he had matters of much greater importance to attend to. This may explain but hardly excuse the remarkable manner in which he expressed his support, which goes so deeply into the heart of the matter that only extensive quotation will do justice to it.

During many of the sessions of the committee there was, and perhaps could be, no dialogue. The anti-vaccinationists had always denied the right of the state to intervene in matters of health between parent and child, and played down the dangers of smallpox; the vaccinationists stressed the dangers of smallpox, and played down both the dangers of 'cow-poxing' and the rights of individuals, for whom, even when their fears were obviously genuine, albeit misguided, Simon could not disguise his disgust. It was on the fourth day of his appearance before the committee, during an exchange with Jacob Bright, that the knives began to flash.

Q I notice in the course of your examination that you have spoken in terms of extreme contempt of your opponents; is it because you think them ignorant and unscientific?

A If your reference is to the anti-vaccination agitators, I think some of them ignorant, and I think others of them dishonest.[7]

Q The extreme contempt which you show for your opponents of course must be based upon the belief on your part that the advantage of vaccination is so self-evident that only an idiot probably could resist it?

A So far as the question is one of intelligence, that is about my opinion.[8]

Q That being so, does it not seem to you a somewhat extraordinary thing that we should require compulsory laws and cumulative fines and imprisonments, in order to make men of common sense and ordinary observing powers accept vaccination?

A The common sense of the public is fairly illustrated by the fact that among the educated classes pretty nearly every one is vaccinated. Among the less educated classes there is a great deal of procrastination, and the main object of the compulsory law is to conquer that difficulty: to conquer indolence and apathy.[9]

Q Then you approve of putting men into prison if they will not be vaccinated contrary to their own belief of the advantages of vaccination?

A I should not myself put it quite in that way. I should regret very much that a person were imprisoned on account of his refusal to have his child vaccinated; it would be to me personally, if I were a magistrate, a very painful necessity to have to send a man to prison under such circumstances; but he is not sent to prison for not having his child vaccinated: he is sent to prison for not obeying the law of his country; and if the judgment of Parliament, the final judgment of the Legislature, is not to be binding on crotchety people in this matter, so immensely important as it is for the public health, no law can be binding.[10]

This reply was at the same time plausible but to some extent specious. A man had been sent to prison for disobeying an order; the order required him to have his child vaccinated; he had not had his child vaccinated; ergo, whatever the ostensible reason, he had been sent to prison for not having his child vaccinated. Section 31 of the Vaccination Act was repeatedly described as 'a remedial measure', that is to say, a legal device to secure what had not been, because in the last resort it could not be, secured by existing legislation. Every parent understood this; the echo of the cane-wielding pedagogue down the ages – 'this hurts me more than it is hurting you' – served merely to emphasize the nature of the insult:

Q You are in favour of something like the present law of compulsion, because as you say there is a great deal of apathy and procrastination?

A Yes.[11]

Q But it is a more important question, is it not, that [whether] compulsion should be exercised not upon those who are apathetic, but upon those who are opposed to vaccination altogether?

A I feel the great difficulty of dealing with crotchety people. I suppose that it is a difficulty that lies in all law making, that you may find people who when they are only very conceited and crotchety, fancy themselves conscientious [...] I wish there were a good loophole for them. I think that the law would be very well quit of them. If it were a case only concerning the parent himself, by all means let the parent go, I would say; but it does not concern only the parent himself, and the State has to judge according to all the evidence which is before it whether vaccination is really such a safeguard to the child's life that the parent ought not to be legally allowed to leave the duty unfulfilled of giving the child that safeguard.[12]

The summary dismissal of 'conscientious' parents as conceited and crotchety prompted Candlish to probe Simon's attitude more deeply. He had said that some opponents of vaccination were 'ignorant' and some 'dishonest'; did he think that the imputation of a corrupt motive was relevant and would help the inquiry?

A I dare say that members of the committee have had before them various sheets of paper making statements against vaccination which are unquestionably dishonest, and which probably every member of the committee would know for himself to be dishonest statements. I hold a bundle of them in my hand, and if it were worth going into such rubbish, they could easily be shown to be dishonest.[13]

Q May there, in your view, be an intelligent, honest opinion against the protectiveness of vaccination?

A No, not if in 'intelligent' you include 'informed', and if by 'opinion' you mean judgment as distinguished from feeling. My meaning, not put offensively, is, that the protectiveness of vaccination is proved by such incontestable facts that no intelligent person, informed of the facts, and weighing them without prejudice, could doubt it.[14]

The doubts, to use no stronger word, expressed by many opponents of vaccination reflected not simply disbelief in its protectiveness but also deep-seated fear of its capacity to inflict unpredictable consequences, a topic on which Simon had also plenty to say, but which must remain for the time being in abeyance.

The select committee, given a question to consider, and having sought advice and opinion from all quarters, came up with a terse answer, or series of answers:

That the cow-pox offers if not an absolute yet a very great protection against an attack of small-pox, and an almost absolute protection against death from that disease.

That if the operation be performed with due regard to the health of the person vaccinated, and with proper precautions in obtaining and using the vaccine lymph, there need be no apprehension that vaccination will injure health or communicate any disease.

That small-pox, unchecked by vaccination, is one of the most terrible and destructive of diseases, as regards the danger of infection, the proportion of deaths among those attacked, and the permanent injury to the survivors; and therefore,

That it is the duty of the State to endeavour to secure the careful vaccination of the whole population.

If the report had stopped there it could truly have been said to have 'carried all before it', but in fact it continued for several pages, demonstrating that far from having been 'rigged' in favour of the pro-vaccination lobby it had paid a great deal of attention to voices counselling caution. Prominent among these was John Candlish who, in his capacity as a witness, had made a statement that his colleagues on the committee had found it inadvisable to ignore. By no means an opponent of vaccination, which he claimed to have had carried out on his own child, he had concentrated on the issue of compulsion which he maintained had not succeeded and could not succeed in achieving its professed aim, the vaccination of the child. The infliction of repeated penalties on the parent was no answer: the child remained unvaccinated. Asked if the law should be made more stringent he argued that it was too stringent already. 'I do not think it is possible in this country to take a child from its parents by violence and have it vaccinated. I know of no other compulsion than taking the child by force [...] I think that no House of Commons would dare to sanction such legislation.'[15]

Whatever the views of individual members the committee as a whole bowed to the inevitable. For the kind of parents 'who from carelessness or forgetfulness delay to protect their children until driven to the vaccine station by panic fear of an epidemic' there could be no objection to a compulsory law; by definition they had no objection to vaccination. There remained the parents – 'very few in number' – who believed that vaccination would harm their children. They might be crotchety, or ill-informed, but if a parent disobeyed two notices or orders the presumption was that he would continue to be 'contumacious', as the official view had it; and since no amount of prosecution was likely to induce him to change his mind there was no point in continuing to harass him. Not only was nothing gained by a long contest with the convictions of the parent; there was the further question of what a later age would call 'public relations':

> When the State, in attempting to fulfil its duty, finds it necessary to disregard the wish of the parent it is most important to secure the support of public opinion, and as your Committee cannot recommend that a policeman should be empowered to take a baby from its mother to the vaccine station, a measure which would only be justified by an extreme necessity, they would recommend that whenever in any case two penalties or one full penalty have been imposed upon a parent the magistrate should not impose any further penalty in respect of the same child.

It had been suggested that the parent's declaration of belief that vaccination was injurious might be pleaded against any penalty, but this would be a step too far and make the law a dead letter. 'Prosecutions would soon cease and the children of many apathetic and neglectful parents would be left unvaccinated, as well as the children of the few opponents of vaccination.'

The concession made by this proposal could only be viewed as a victory for common sense; even Simon, giving evidence, had grudgingly agreed with the suggestion, emanating from Candlish, that two penalties 'would fully answer the purpose as regards the mass of the population'. Nobody was rash or unkind enough to inquire what he would propose to do about the rest.

Perhaps feeling that it had conceded enough to anti-vaccinationist sentiment the committee redressed the balance by proposing to grant to the vaccination department a measure that it had long hankered after. All earlier legislation had in one important respect been permissive: it had been left to guardians to decide whether or not to prosecute a defaulting parent. The unwillingness of some boards to embark on proceedings had left objectors a loophole by which to avoid fines or imprisonment and relieve the ratepayers of a further financial burden. One proposal to take a contested case to the court of appeal had been withdrawn at a late stage because of the likely expense involved. The committee dealt summarily with the problem: 'By section 28 the guardians of every union or parish may appoint an officer to promote vaccination and to prosecute offenders against the Act [...] Your committee recommend that this appointment be made obligatory on the guardians.' The 'vaccination officer', as he would be known, would take over from the registrar much of the paperwork, including keeping the vaccination register and the issuing of certificates, that had been such a burden and in consequence so badly neglected.

Once again Simon's retrospective assessment is worth noting:

> the final report of the Committee [...] gave the Committee's unequivocal verdict against accusers who had challenged the inquiry. It proclaimed afresh to the world the powerful protective value as well as the almost certain innocuousness of the properly formed vesicle and expressed approval of the principle of the Act which had made infantine vaccination compulsory.[16]

A footnote adds that 'the House of Commons did not accept the Committee's recommendation to provide against cumulative penalties': a comment that suggests that economy with the truth is not a modern phenomenon.

With a Bill in preparation incorporating the committee's mutually agreed adjustments to the law the vaccination department, which had surrendered little and gained much, could rest content. For all but the most refractory parents, escape from the net of the Vaccination Act was now almost impossible. Moreover it seemed that elsewhere in the system the most irksome hindrance to the work of the department was about to be removed.

From the earliest days of state provision of free vaccination there had been, as discussed above, great controversy over the decision to hand the responsibility for operating the service to the boards of guardians set up to administer the Poor Law Act of 1834. The two functions were mutually incompatible. Dissatisfaction had hardened to something like open hostility with the appointment of Simon as Chief Medical Officer to the Privy Council in the late 1850s, and the opening of his campaign for reform of the quantity and quality of vaccination, which brought a clash of interests into the open. Simon, on behalf of the Privy Council, prescribed how and by whom public vaccination should be carried out, and laid down agreed standards of proficiency, but control of the contracts under which public vaccinators were recruited, supervised and paid remained with the Poor Law Board, which was dilatory, sometimes to the point of obstruction, in carrying out the recommendations of the medical experts. In particular the Poor Law Board, which had no medical practitioners on its staff, took no responsibility for a key area of the whole vaccination system, the maintenance of an adequate and satisfactory supply of lymph, through the arm-to-arm method.

By 1871 it seemed that the conflict might at last be on the point of resolution. The government had decided that a number of hitherto independent departments, with often ill-defined and overlapping responsibilities, should be brought together in a new department. A Bill was introduced for the creation of a Local Government Board, which duly came into existence in August with, among its component parts, much of the medical department of the Privy Council, whose staff, instead of acquiring full responsibility for public vaccination, found themselves part of a large organization in which questions of health took a low priority.

Three years later, in response to some extravagant claims by Robert Lowe concerning alleged improvements made by himself and other members of Gladstone's government, the *British Medical Journal* put these developments in a different perspective:

> Read by the light of sober facts the Government has detached the Sanitary Department of the Privy Council from its former connections and has subordinated it to the destitution department [i.e. the former Poor Law Board, now extinguished]. It has placed over it a minister who has obstinately and scornfully refused to recognise it as a department, and who has persistently treated it as a subordinate part of the organisation for the relief of destitution. Mr Stansfield has deliberately slighted and snubbed the officers of the Health Department [...] and lest he should be compelled to recognise Mr Simon as the head of a department, he has studiously avoided consulting him on all important occasions.[17]

The consequence for Simon was catastrophic. As he wrote years later,

> The Privy Council's powers and duties of a medical kind had not all been made over to the new Department: so, in respect of some of the matters for which I had been Medical Officer of the Privy Council I remained in their Lordships' service: but in respect of those which related to local government [including] the superintendence of vaccination [...] my office was [now] 'attached to and under the control of the Local Government Board'.[18]

No man can serve two masters. Simon struggled on, deprived of most of his status and powers, until 1876 and then retired, a broken and embittered man. He was succeeded by Seaton who, worn out by more than forty years in the cause of vaccination, died in 1880. In spite of the calculated personal snub to Simon which the Local Government Act delivered, the passage of the Vaccination Act of the same year (1874) completed the edifice of compulsion that he and his colleagues had laboured to construct; but even this success was not achieved without an episode that had the most far-reaching consequences.

The Bill setting out the amendments that were to be incorporated into the main Act made the purpose of the exercise clear from the start. Section 5 stipulated that it would in future be obligatory for guardians to appoint 'vaccination officers', whose status in the new hierarchy was crisply defined. 'The Poor Law Board shall have the same powers with respect to guardians and vaccination officers in matters relating to vaccination as they have with respect to guardians and officers of guardians in matters relating to the relief of the poor, and may make rules, orders and regulations accordingly'. Subsequent sections dealt with the transfer of duties and responsibilities from registrars to vaccination officers. Relegated to the tenth position, almost as an after-thought, was the section dealing with the vexed question of cumulative penalties, which had occupied so much of the select committee's time:

> after the commencement of this Act no parent of a child shall be liable to be convicted for neglecting to take [...] such child to be vaccinated if either
>
> a) He has been previously adjudged to pay the full penalty of twenty shillings for any such offence with respect to such child, or
>
> b) He has been previously twice adjudged to pay any penalty for any such offence for such child.

During a brief debate in the Commons to consider the Bill as amended in committee, Sir Michael Hicks-Beach argued that the clause, if passed, would 'make the House stultify itself' by revoking a decision that it had come to in 1867, while at the same time it maintained the reasoning and opinions that had induced it to arrive at that decision. He did not wish to see a policeman take a baby from its mother but there was an alternative: 'The vaccination authority might be empowered to visit the homes of defaulting parents, and there and then vaccinate the children'.[19]

Defending the clause on behalf of the government Forster said that he had never assisted at a more puzzling investigation, and that members of the select committee had gone into the inquiry entirely opposed to the view that they ultimately adopted. Rejecting Hicks-Beach's bizarre proposal on the ground that nothing would be more likely to excite public opinion against the Act, he hoped the House would adopt what had been the unanimous opinion of the committee.

Hibbert, speaking for the Poor Law authorities, believed the Bill would tend to allay the existing excitement against vaccination, and 'get rid of the societies formed in various parts of the country in opposition to the principle of compulsory vaccination'. The House then passed the Bill in its entirety by 57 votes to 12, and on the following day it went forward to face its last remaining hurdle, the House of Lords.[20]

The government spokesman, Viscount Halifax, having given the almost mandatory recital of the horrors and havoc wrought by smallpox and the inestimable advantages offered by vaccination, clearly expected the Bill to be passed without too much fuss. He was proved wrong. One of their Lordships, Viscount Redesdale, incensed by the paragraph concerning repeated prosecutions which he held, in common with many inside and outside Parliament, would undermine the whole purpose of the Vaccination Acts, had put down an amendment calling for the clause to be withdrawn. Halifax, attempting to ward off the attack, asserted that 'Mr Simon [...] is of opinion that it is unwise to insist upon anything which is not indispensable' but Lord Redesdale could not be dissuaded from dividing the House. There were fifteen peers present: seven voted against the amendment, eight for it, and the Bill in its mutilated state was returned to the Commons.

In normal circumstances the Commons would almost certainly have restored the clause and challenged the Lords to interfere with it again, but the circumstances were not normal. The Lords' rejection of the clause took place on a Friday. Parliament was to be prorogued on Monday, and any Act that had not received the royal assent by then would lapse. The government was anxious not to lose the main part of the Bill, and there was insufficient time for it to be sent back to the Lords in its original form. When the Commons met on Saturday morning Forster, not attempting to conceal his anger, explained the situation.[21] Faced with the impasse the Commons had no alternative. The Bill was given its third reading, minus the disputed clause. Opponents of vaccination could in future, as in the past, be prosecuted *toties quoties*. The vote of one member of the House of Lords had frustrated a reform of the Act that, if passed as the government had intended, would have obviated twenty-five years of antagonism, obstruction and distress. It was probably this event, more than any other, that fuelled the militant phase of the anti-vaccination campaign.

PART II

The Reign of Compulsion

CHAPTER 14

A LOATHSOME VIRUS

As has been noted, condemnation of compulsory vaccination dates from shortly after the passage of the Act of 1853, with the letter from John Gibbs to the President of the Board of Health. Born in Ireland in 1811, Gibbs was described by an acquaintance as 'sagacious, bright, earnest and independent', with a passion for 'such things as made for human welfare and improvement'. He became interested in hydropathy and in particular in its use in cases of smallpox. In later life he made his home in St Leonards, in Sussex. His influential letter to the Board of Health was based on a pamphlet that he had published in 1854 under the title 'Our Medical Liberties'.

'The partisans of compulsory vaccination,' he wrote, 'cast away every gentlemanly feeling, disregard every principle of justice, violate the spirit of freedom, outrage the precepts of Christianity, trample upon common sense, betray their own rights and dearest interests.'[1] After this comprehensive denunciation he took each item in turn and expanded it, occasionally in the repetitive fashion that became one of the continuing characteristics and weaknesses of the whole long campaign.

The compulsory Vaccination Act, he asserted, was

the first direct aggression upon the person of the subject in medical matters which has been attempted in these kingdoms. It invades in the most unexampled manner the liberty of the subject and the sanctity of the home [...] it sets at nought parental responsibility and constrains the parent either to violate his deliberate convictions, and even his religious scruples, or to defy an unjust law.

Why was vaccination held in horror by so many parents and others?

They do not believe that it affords an efficient and assured protection against the invasion of small-pox: they have a natural disgust of transferring to the veins of their children a loathsome virus derived from the blood of a diseased brute and transmitted through they know not how many unhealthy mediums [i.e. by the arm-to-arm method]: they have a dread, a conviction, that other filthy diseases, tending to embitter and shorten life, are frequently transmitted through and by the vaccine virus [a reference to the dread of syphilis] [...] and further they have a conscientious conviction that voluntarily to propagate disease is to fly in the face of God and to violate that precept which says 'Do thyself no harm'. Are such scruples entitled to no respect?

Having supplied the rebellion with its manifesto Gibbs appears to have personally taken little further part in its progress, although other members of his family became closely involved. His health declined and he died in 1875. By that time, after a slow beginning, opposition to compulsion had gathered momentum, coming into prominence first in the north of England, chiefly in Manchester and Leeds.

Among the earliest names to become associated with the campaign was that of Henry Pitman, one of three brothers of whom the second, Isaac, was the inventor of a successful system of shorthand known as phonography, and the third a printer. Henry described his profession as 'lecturer and teacher of phonography' and advertised his availability as an instructor of working men on a variety of topics in fields such as economics, politics and trade unionism.

In 1860 the Co-operative movement, which had been inaugurated in a small way in Rochdale, Lancashire, in 1844, and had spread rapidly through the manufacturing districts, launched a periodical, *The Co-operator*, 'conducted exclusively by working men', price one penny, to instruct the membership in the philosophy and practice of the Co-operative ideal. Like many publications of its kind, carried on in their spare time by men wholly untrained in the profession of journalism, it was well-meaning, passionately earnest and virtually unreadable, and held very little appeal for its intended readers, who ceased to support it, although the second number in July 1860 carried an enthusiastic letter from Henry Pitman. In June 1863 it was announced that Pitman was to become its editor, running it apparently as a private speculation. In spite of the improvements he introduced it continued to languish and plunged him into an almost unending financial predicament, which was not lessened when, as a supporter of the anti-vaccination cause, he virtually hijacked *The Co-operator*, merging it with a weekly publication called *The Anti-Vaccinator* that he had launched in 1869 and turning it into a propaganda medium for anti-vaccination, from which discussion of cooperation was almost entirely banished. This unlikely marriage was dissolved in 1872 and *The Co-operator* went its own way.

Pitman later explained that he and his wife, having had their first children vaccinated in accordance with the law, had come to regard the operation with horror and determined that none of their future children should undergo it. This decision being acted upon duly brought Pitman into conflict with the law, and having passed through the stages of neglecting to have a child vaccinated, then refusing to obey a specific instruction to have the operation performed within seven days, and finally refusing to pay the fine imposed, he was committed to Knutsford House of Correction for fourteen days. He subsequently published a humorous account of his experiences, which showed that as a man of some standing in the community he was treated with greater deference than was shown in later years to humbler dissidents in other gaols.[2] His fine was paid by a friend, Hugh Birley, MP for Manchester, and he was released, somewhat to his disappointment, to carry on *The Anti-Vaccinator*.

Among his collaborators was a prominent figure in the academic and literary world, Professor Francis Newman, the younger brother of Cardinal Henry Newman, and as little like him in temperament and achievement as it would seem possible to be. Recalled by an acquaintance as 'a vegetarian, a total abstainer, and enemy of tobacco, vaccination and vivisection', and elsewhere as 'a proponent of polymathic unorthodoxy in, among other things, the pronunciation of Latin, millenialism, theology and Arabian lexicography', his acquaintance with Pitman began in 1869 when, having read in a periodical that 'a horrible virus is extending itself in the blood of the English People [and] it is clearly possible that much of the evil is from vaccination', he applied to join the recently formed Anti-Compulsory Vaccination League. In a letter introducing himself to Pitman he condemned the principle of vaccination as 'untenable' and laid particular blame on those who, like Florence Nightingale, took for granted that 'children *must* have measles and other diseases', which led him to

> put the finger on the weak spot of the doctors, alike of the body politic and of the individual body; Instead of saying – 'There ought to be no poverty, no disease, our public regulations must never be allowed to *cause* it', their sole question is – How to palliate it? [...] In pressing on the Legislature compulsory vaccination, instead of pressing to remove all causes of small-pox, they assume that small-pox does not spring out of removable causes [...] But to enact and enforce vaccination with something or other, when the

legislators cannot enforce that the virus shall be pure of its kind, is so indefensible, that it might seem a mere representation would lead to repeal, or lead ministers to suspend the Act during enquiry.[3]

He was, as might be expected, a bitter opponent of the compulsory Act on moral as well as medical grounds: 'To enact a medical creed or command a medical process is usurpation – not legitimate legislation, even viewed from the scientific side'. Viewed on the side of freedom it was a horrible atrocity: 'What can be more shocking than when vaccination has killed one child of a family to compel the parents to yield up a second child to the same treatment? What is it but murder?' As a practical contribution to the campaign against the act, Newman gave Pitman financial assistance in launching *The Anti-Vaccinator* and subscribed to the various associations that at one time or another were founded to promote the struggle against compulsion.

Two other active campaigners in the early days were the Revd William Hume-Rothery and his wife Mary, the daughter of the radical politician Joseph Hume. William in particular was typical of the *post hoc ergo propter hoc* school of anti-vaccinationists. Whatever ailments a child suffered from, even death, would often be ascribed by its parents to its having been vaccinated, however demonstrably improbable any connection between the two events. Hume-Rothery would accept these protestations at face value, making no attempt to obtain independent medical opinion. One of the campaign's *Vaccination Tracts* reprinted a list of alleged 'Cases of injury and death produced by vaccination' collected in one Lancashire town with a view to their being presented before the select committee, which refused to receive them, not surprisingly in view of their style and content:

Martha Alice Jackson, daughter of James Jackson, of Stoneyfield Rochdale, vaccinated when three weeks old, by Dr. Booth, public vaccinator. About nine days after vaccination it broke out of a most loathsome disease, designated by the medical attendant, Dr. Morris, as a very bad case of syphilis, caused, the medical man said, by vaccination. It suffered dreadfully until seven months old, and then died a most pitiable object.

Robert Henry Fielding, son of Thomas Fielding, Radcliffe Street, Rochdale, was vaccinated when four months old. The arm immediately began to swell towards the fingers, then across the chest and down the right arm, which was very much swollen, and after death the arm burst. The child died one month after vaccination. The medical attendant told the father that vaccination had killed the child. It died January 1870.

Edwin Kershaw, son of Emmanuel Kershaw, Oldham Road, Rochdale, was vaccinated when five months old, in January 1870, and died a fortnight after being vaccinated. The arm of the child was so bad that it began to mortify and burst before death. It was a most deplorable object. Dr. Booth, the public vaccinator, performed the operation of vaccination. Dr. Morris, the medical attendant, certified the cause of death as being vaccination.

Died, December 10th, 1871, after much suffering, Robert Arthur Batchelder of 59 Clarendon Street, Harrow Road, aged four months. The child was vaccinated by Dr. Graves on the 27th November, being then in perfect health. Seven days after, the skin and countenance became yellow, the matter which came from the vaccination punctures was deep yellow, and stained the linen. The child was in great agony, *and lost its voice from incessant screaming*, getting no sleep day nor night. His was evidently a case of jaundice produced by pyaemia, or blood-poisoning, the direct result of vaccination.[4]

A more formidable anti-vaccinationist was James John Garth Wilkinson, friend of many distinguished men of letters and himself a prolific author. He had set out to train as a doctor but had found the atmosphere of early nineteenth-century dissecting rooms and operating theatres more than he could take, and had turned instead to the practice of homoeopathy, which produced a sufficiently satisfactory livelihood to enable him to occupy premises in fashionable Wimpole Street. A man of strong religious convictions he became a devout follower of the Swedish mystic Swedenborg, whose writings exercised a profound influence on the life and thought of a group of the most articulate opponents of vaccination. Mrs Hume-Rothery, Isaac Pitman – the brother of Henry – and William White, of whom more later, were disciples of Swedenborg, although not in most cases involved in the sectarian politics and squabbles that disfigured much of the early history of the Church of the New Jerusalem.

Emanuel Swedenborg (1688–1772) had progressed from being a gifted engineer and scientist to the study of the mechanisms of the natural world and its relation to and interaction with the spiritual world, and finally into realms of mysticism where his claims to spiritual experience strained the credulity of all but his most dedicated followers. The titles of three of his early works (translated from the original Latin) illustrate the sequence and development of his search for the physical basis of the psyche:

1. *The Principia: or the First Principles of Natural Things; being New Attempts Towards a Philosophical Explanation of the Elementary World.*

2. *The Philosophy of the Infinite: or Outlines of a Philosophical Argument on the Infinite, and the Final Cause of Creation; and on the Intercourse between the Soul and the Body.*

3. *The Economy of the Animal Kingdom: considered Anatomically, Physically and Philosophically.*

A Swedish authority points out that the English title of the last-named work is 'utterly misleading' to the modern reader. 'Not one word of it means what it seems to say', because the translation follows too slavishly the Latin title. 'Animal' in this connection is derived from 'anima', the Latin for 'soul'. The title should be 'The Organization (or Government) of the Soul's Kingdom', that is, the body.[5]

It would scarcely seem possible that the anatomical and physiological metaphors of an eighteenth-century mystic should have more than a passing interest for mid- and late nineteenth-century intellectuals, and White, at least, who laboured to summarize and expound them, found the job infinitely taxing. Yet in 1845 the Swedenborg Association was formed for the express purpose of disinterring some of these works from the dusty Latin in which they had lain buried for a century and reissuing them in English translation, in which form they almost immediately suffered, as White put it, 'the pain of a second death'.

One of the volunteers who undertook this immense and ultimately fruitless task was Garth Wilkinson. He seems to have found the labour of translation less stifling and unrewarding than White found ploughing through the result, and one of the volumes earned him lavish praise from an unexpected source. Shortly after its appearance it came to the notice of the American poet, essayist and philosopher Ralph Waldo Emerson, who found in it just what he was looking for. One of his own best-known publications consists of the texts of a series of lectures on *Representative Men*, each devoted to a study of a figure outstanding in his own walk of life: Plato, Shakespeare, Montesquieu, Goethe, Napoleon, among others. Having a strong tendency to a mystical interpretation of nature and human experience, Emerson took as one of his subjects 'Swedenborg the mystic', but as he got to grips with the subject much of his admiration for this representative man evaporated. Strangely it was Swedenborg's matter-of-fact relation of his own mystical experiences that most offended Emerson: 'When he mounts into heaven I do not hear its language. A man should not tell me that he has walked among the angels [...] Strange, scholastic, didactic, passionless, bloodless man [...] he has no sympathy [...] [he] is disagreeably wise and with all his accumulated gifts, paralyses and repels.'

At this point Emerson might have been expected either to look around for a mystic whose personality and message had more to offer him or to abandon the realm of mysticism altogether, but his attention was drawn to those earlier scientific works, especially *The Economy of the Animal Kingdom*, 'a book of wonderful merit [...] one of those books which by the sustained dignity of thinking, is an honour to the human race [...] The grandeur of the topic makes the grandeur of the style.' He could not of course find his way through Swedenborg's turgid, meandering Latin but the work had now been translated into English by 'Mr. Wilkinson, a philosophic critic, with a co-equal vigour of understanding and imagination comparable only to Lord Bacon'. High praise indeed.

The aspect of Swedenborg's work that links it to the campaign against vaccination arises out of his investigation of 'the Intercourse between the Soul and the Body', which led him to concentrate his attention on the blood whose composition and function he describes in the highly charged but totally undisciplined prose that characterizes his vast output: 'Whatever exists in the body pre-exists in the blood'; 'The blood is the complex of all things that exist in the world'; 'it would appear as if all things were created for the purpose of administering to the composition and continual renewal of the blood'; 'every globule of blood has both a soul and a body, and what is true of all the parts is also true of the whole that lives in the blood'. Through Wilkinson's efforts, perhaps, something of Swedenborg's concept of the blood and its universal significance communicated itself to the anti-vaccinationists for whom, even more than for those of Jenner's time, one of the principal horrors of vaccination was the contamination of the blood of their newborn children by the injection into it of matter from a diseased animal. 'The blood' runs like a refrain through much anti-vaccinationist literature and rhetoric.

In addition to his professional work as a homoeopath and the immense burden of translating Swedenborg, Wilkinson's conscience was, as he put it, 'assailed' in 1865 by the Countess De Noailles (Lady Mount Temple) who induced him to look into the subject of vaccination. His first impression, as conveyed to the Countess, was that 'Vaccination is an infinitesimal affair: its reform will come with greater reforms'.[6] He had in fact performed the operation on himself and others. Further study changed his mind: 'As forced upon every British Cradle, I see it as a Monster instead of a poisonous Midge [...] As a Destroyer of the Honesty and Humanity of Medicine, which is through it a deeply degraded Profession [...] abolishing the last hope and resort of races, the newborn soundness of the Human Body.' As a result of this conversion Wilkinson poured out a stream of polemical works on the subject of the supposed evils of vaccination. Prominent among them were a series of fourteen *Vaccination Tracts* which supplied campaigners for the anti-vaccination cause with the basis of much of their own beliefs and assertions.

The ostensible source of the tracts, which appeared anonymously, was William Young, a pharmaceutical chemist whose work as editor Wilkinson took over on Young's death, but there seems little doubt that they all owed much of their vigour and passion chiefly to Wilkinson himself. Although they appeared fairly early in the campaign, over a period of years from 1877, they incorporated most of the arguments that sustained it during the two decades when it was at its height.

The early tracts were occupied largely by cases, similar to those quoted above, of young children who, having been vaccinated, died within a short (or sometimes a fairly long) time later. The official verdict was frequently 'erysipelas', a skin disease that the parents and the anti-vaccinationists insisted was caused by vaccination, whereas the authorities maintained that there was and could be no connection.

Another staple element of the tracts, and of anti-vaccination propaganda in general, was a vast accumulation of statistics designed to demonstrate that vaccination was at best ineffective and at worst a killer in its own right. The war of statistics was waged without respite or scruple for upwards of two decades, each side routinely dismissing the other's ammunition as flawed or downright fraudulent.

Tract number 7, largely the work of Wilkinson, was a polemic entitled 'Vaccination a sign of the Decay of the Political and Medical Conscience of the Country' and drew heavily on Swedenborg's *Animal Kingdom* with its emphasis on the significance of the purity of the blood ('Vaccination mingles in a communion of blood the taints of the community'):

Poison inserted into the blood of infants is fivefold: *First poison*, the matter of vaccine disease itself. *Second poison*, the occasional and constitutional diseases of the cow from which the matter is derived [...] *Third poison*, the vaccine disease of the human being. *Fourth poison*, the occasional and constitutional diseases of the child and family from which the matter was taken [by the arm-to-arm method]. And *Fifth poison*, the gathered taints of all the children through whose systems the matter has passed since it left the cow.[7]

One of the most significant tracts, number 9, listed many examples of multiple prosecutions, fines and imprisonments imposed upon 'contumacious' parents. Tables showed as many as 44 fines inflicted on one individual (in some cases the fines imposed on poor offenders were probably paid by wealthy sympathizers). Questions asked from time to time in Parliament resulted in the publication of similar, official, statistics. Long and ostensibly plausible accounts, included in the tract, described the brutal and humiliating treatment suffered by parents whose intransigence was punished by a prison sentence.

The conclusion of the final tract (number 14) was that vaccination was 'a universal force exerted upon the nation's life. No other legal force is so general. It is the largest net of compulsion into which the population is swept by Government power.'

CHAPTER 15

A CRUEL AND DEGRADING IMPOSTURE

Among the most prominent opponents of vaccination were two members of the medical profession, one more eminent than the other. Edgar Crookshank, Professor of Comparative Pathology and Bacteriology and Fellow of King's College, London, wrote a *History and Pathology of Vaccination* in two volumes (1889). The Preface to the first volume described how, following some investigations into an outbreak of cowpox, he became convinced that

> the commonly accepted descriptions of the nature and origins of Cow Pox were purely theoretical [...] I gradually became so deeply impressed with the small amount of knowledge possessed by practitioners concerning Cow Pox, and other sources of Vaccine Lymph, and with the conflicting teachings and opinions of leading authorities, in both the medical and veterinary professions, that I determined to investigate the subject for myself.

The essence of Crookshank's argument against vaccination was that the power of conferring immunity to smallpox, claimed for cowpox by disciples of Jenner, was a fallacy because what was injected under the guise of cowpox was in fact smallpox. The origins of this controversy lay in the earliest period when, with supplies of cowpox very scarce for lack of suitable outbreaks to draw on, some confusion had occurred over a consignment of alleged cowpox despatched by Jenner from London to a colleague in the country. Detractors claimed that, whether by accident or from lack of scruple, Jenner had in fact supplied his friend with smallpox lymph, and that since the material in question had formed the basis for thousands of 'ingrafting' operations carried out from arm to arm right down to Crookshank's own time, any immunity ascribed to cowpox should really be ascribed to the effects of smallpox. This theory was revived in recent times but has been investigated by Baxby who finds no basis for it.[1]

Crookshank's general conclusion as a result of his investigation was that the medical profession had been misled by Jenner, by his biographer, Baron, by the Reports of the National Vaccine Establishment and by a want of knowledge concerning the nature of cowpox, horsepox and other sources of 'vaccine lymph':

the pathology of [cowpox] and its nature and affinities have not been made the subject of practical study for nearly half a century. We have submitted instead to purely theoretical teaching and have been led to regard vaccination as inoculation of the human subject with a *benign disease of the cow*, whereas the viruses in use have been derived from several distinct and severe diseases in different animals.[2]

He ended with a broadside aimed at most of the members of his profession:

Unfortunately a belief in the efficiency of vaccination has been so enforced in the education of the medical practitioner that it is hardly probable that the futility of the practice will be acknowledged in our generation, though nothing would more redound to the credit of the profession and give evidence of the advance made in pathology and sanitary science. It is more probable that when, by means of notification and isolation, Small Pox is kept under control vaccination will disappear from practice and will retain only a historic interest.[3]

Crookshank's views were inevitably ridiculed by his professional colleagues, who were also incensed by his support for an early opponent of vaccination who had invited his readers to reflect on 'the excessive filth and nastiness which must unavoidably mix with the milk in the infected dairy of cows, and the corrupt and unsalubrious state of their produce'. Crookshank himself reported the 'filth and nastiness' of a Wiltshire farm where cowpox had broken out, and had advocated the placing of the disease under the Contagious Diseases (Animals) Act.

For these misdemeanours, which struck at the root of the whole vaccination philosophy, Crookshank was treated with extraordinary aggression and incivility when he gave evidence to the Royal Commission of 1889. Under the bombardment he retracted some of his views on the nature and efficiency of cowpox, but was subsequently vindicated in part when his views (shared with other partisans) on the use of notification and isolation of smallpox cases became accepted as standard practice in the control of the disease.

Crookshank's views may have been anathema to his professional colleagues but they were welcomed with the greatest enthusiasm by his fellow anti-vaccinationists, as were, with much less justification, those of another polemicist and renegade from the ranks of orthodoxy, Charles Creighton. Creighton's career was summed up in the obituary notice, written by his friend Professor William Bulloch, that appeared in the *Lancet* in 1927: 'England [has lost] her most learned medical scholar of the 19th century, although it cannot be forgotten that some of his opinions were the subject of such criticism that he ceased to be felt as a power in the medical world.'

A Scot, born in Peterhead, Creighton studied medicine at Aberdeen and Edinburgh universities. His *magnum opus* was *The History of Epidemics in Britain* (two volumes, 1894), which when reprinted in recent times was held still to possess considerable value. When the original version appeared, however, he had already destroyed his credibility with a series of publications, for one of which a distinguished member of the medical profession felt it necessary, even after the passage of thirty or forty years, to apologize on behalf of the profession.

Creighton's problem, his obituarist wrote, was that 'he simply could not acclimatise himself to modern [i.e. nineteenth-century] theories of disease. He belonged medically to another age: he lived in a world of miasms and effluvia rather than of particulate contagion in the form of bacteria.' The two books that undermined his reputation were *Illustrations of the Unconscious Memory of Disease* (1885) and *The Natural History of Cowpox and Vaccinal Syphilis* (1886). The combined message of the two works can be expressed briefly: there was no connection between cowpox and smallpox, but there was a connection, derived by way of the process of 'unconscious memory' (of disease), between cowpox and the great pox, i.e. syphilis, of which theory one critic wrote that 'nothing in the history of pathology can be more absurd'.

The corollary of these doctrines, which Creighton did not hesitate to point out, was that the notion of 'cowpoxing', i.e. vaccination, as a prophylactic against smallpox was a fallacy. It was therefore surprising that he should have been invited to contribute an article on 'Vaccination' to the ninth edition of the *Encyclopaedia Britannica* which appeared in 1888 (in spite of the sequence of publication dates, which places the article later than the books, Creighton told the Royal Commission of 1889 that it was while writing the article that he was led to look into the whole subject, with of course his unexpected conclusions). The article, while drawing on his vast and undisputed knowledge of the history of smallpox, epidemics, and so on, restated his views on vaccination, and would have finally sealed his fate even if he had not followed it a year later with *Jenner and Vaccination*. He had already proclaimed his conviction that Jenner was mistaken: that cowpox was not, as Jenner believed, 'variolae vaccinae' (smallpox of the cow); and that cowpox did not protect against smallpox. He now delivered an astonishing diatribe against Jenner, both as a man and a member of the medical profession, which, in the words of a modern scholar, 'added the crime of iconoclasm to mere eccentricity'.

In a brief summary of Jenner's career before the publication of his *Inquiry* Creighton attempted to demolish or cast cynical doubt on most of what had hitherto been taken as creditable to him. Specimens believed to show Jenner's skill at dissecting and preparation were probably not his own work but were bought for him; the research he had done for Hunter, the great naturalist, consisted of 'a few meagre observations'; his discovery and description of the remarkable process by which the young cuckoo takes possession of its host's nest, although accepted as reliable by all ornithologists, was 'a tissue of inconsistencies and absurdities'. As for Jenner's views on the relationship between cowpox and smallpox: 'It was just because Jenner had no profound sense of the empirical realities that he went blundering into visionary nonsense in the first instance and at length into systematic mystification and chicane'.

This was the substance of Creighton's whole charge against Jenner – that he was an unscrupulous fraud:

If the [medical] profession and the public had been permitted to know (at the time) all that they now know [...] they would probably have found out Jenner to be the vain, imaginative, loose-thinking person that he was by nature, and they might have so acted as to prevent him from becoming the impostor and shuffler that the course of events made him.[4]

In a chapter headed 'The Pox, the Small-Pox and the Cow-Pox' Creighton asserted that 'The single bond connecting cowpox with smallpox was the occurrence of the word "pox" in each name'. Cowpox, according to Creighton, was 'fancifully represented as an amulet or charm against small-pox by the idle gossip of credulous persons who listened only to the jingle of names [...] It is difficult to acquit Jenner of recklessness, or of culpable laxity, even in the very inception of his idea.' In the succeeding chapter Jenner's *Inquiry* received the same caustic treatment, which was later extended to the entire medical profession for having allowed itself to be so easily bamboozled by him.

The significance of these otherwise long-forgotten polemics, published when anti-vaccination already had a history of three decades or more, is that Creighton was readily hailed, as Bulloch testified, by the anti-vaccinationists as a recruit to their ranks, although a more recent researcher doubts whether he belonged there. The medical profession by contrast 'treated him with disdain and obloquy [...] and if he was ever referred to at all it was only as "Creighton the Anti-vaccinator"'. The irony is that among his other literary labours was his translation from the German of Hirsch's highly regarded *Handbook of Geographical and Historical Pathology* (1883) in which, discussing the 'Influence of Vaccination on the Prevalence of Smallpox', Hirsch wrote:

> the achievement of Jenner was at once a turning point in the history of smallpox and a new era in the physical welfare of mankind [...] it can only be folly or stupidity that would seek nowadays to minimize or to question the immortal merits of Jenner [or to attempt] to discredit vaccination...[5]

One pictures Creighton gritting his teeth as his self-imposed task required him to convict himself of folly or stupidity.

Creighton later gave evidence to the Royal Commission on Vaccination and had to stand up to some very rough handling by a predictably hostile and contemptuous panel of inquisitors who submitted his writings and beliefs to the same searching criticism as he had meted out to Jenner. Two questions, and his answers, said it all:

> Q (5430) Will you kindly tell me whether in your opinion vaccination affords any protection against smallpox?
>
> A I have been desirous of avoiding the broad question but as you have asked it I suppose I am bound to answer it. In my opinion it affords none.
>
> Q (5126) [...]your conclusion from the early history of vaccination is that it is a delusion and an imposture which has been fostered by the medical profession and which had no other foundation?
>
> A [quoting from one of his own works] [...] 'The anti-vaccinationists are those who have found some motive for scrutinizing the evidence, generally the very human motive of vaccinal injuries

or fatalities in their own families or in those of their neighbours. Whatever their motive they have scrutinized the evidence to some purpose: they have mastered nearly the whole case; they have knocked the bottom out of a grotesque superstition.'

In suggesting that vaccination might be looked upon as a 'delusion' and an 'imposture' the questioner may perhaps have been unconsciously or deliberately prompted by the title of the work that more comprehensively than any other put the case against compulsory vaccination: William White's *The Story of a Great Delusion*, published in 1885.

White, like Garth Wilkinson, was a follower of Swedenborg, and wrote his *Life and Work* in two volumes, a task that he found daunting: '[He] is not an author to be read through [...] most who make the attempt find themselves yawning or asleep before they get far.' This did not diminish his respect for the man and his spiritual vision. 'My admiration of Swedenborg is wholly intellectual', he declared:

What he relates [of his experience of the spiritual world] may be true or untrue: I have no means of judging [...] Other details I read and credit. Why? Because they seem consonant with such experience as I have had in this world, or because they seem orderly growths of the laws of the Spiritual World [...] Yet this faith I hold modestly, subject to correction, knowing how easy it is to be mistaken.[6]

There could hardly be a greater contrast between this diffident modesty and the dogmatic, aggressive onslaught of *The Great Delusion*, a compendium of all the arguments against compulsory vaccination, an anthology of texts from the preceding generations of anti-vaccinationists (useful but unfortunately not always giving their sources), and a bitter assault, in the vein of Creighton, on the work and character of Jenner. It is a long book, and it is amusing to find the author who complained that Swedenborg was 'iterative' claiming for his own book: 'I am explicit to iteration because the truth is not recognized and may be accounted incredible'.

After an introduction in general terms White assembles the arguments put forward in the early eighteenth century against the practice of inoculation for smallpox (variolation) and shows how closely some of them anticipated the opposition to vaccination a century later. He traces the development of inoculation from the costly and complicated process of the early days through to the greatly simplified system popularized, at least among the better-off classes, by Sutton, Dimsdale and others. Arriving at Jenner he proceeds to dismantle the claims made in the *Inquiry* and in Jenner's later defence and expansion of his theory.

Here he is at times on uncomfortably firm ground. There had always been debate, sometimes furious, concerning Jenner's claims for cowpox in relation to smallpox; most of it, conducted within the limits of what was known about both diseases, is now of little more than academic interest. What the medical profession knew in those days was at best little more than rudimentary, and much of what it thought it knew was, from a theoretical point of view, false or at best misleading. No one could explain satisfactorily, for example, why a survivor of an attack of smallpox was most unlikely ever to experience another one, or why cowpox might prevent an attack of smallpox; the nature of the body's immune system was not even suspected, let alone understood, for another century and more. Most physicians were probably content to echo, if only in private, Frewen (1749): 'the powers of nature and the true causes of things are too difficult to be resolved, and will probably remain a secret with the great Giver and Disposer of things, whose mysterious rule and order of providence is beyond the reach of human comprehension'. From this agnostic starting point it was an easy step to a pragmatic approach to the practice of medicine:

> Some things, however difficult to be accounted for, appear notwithstanding manifestly plain to our discerning senses – why the same particles of infecting matter, infused into different bodies, should be productive of different kinds of Small-Pox, we can no more account for than why we were made with such and such different features and complexions.[7]

Eighteen years later another physician, Langton, admitted candidly, 'How an infection can [...] remain suspended, so as to give the Small-Pox to one who has never had it, and not to one who has, or what the disposition of habit, or the modification of the miasmata, are wholly inexplicable'.[8] In 1796, the year in which Jenner carried out his first experimental inoculation of cowpox, Woodville, in his *History of the Inoculation of the Small-Pox*, admitted that '[n]o satisfactory reason has yet been given why an inoculated Small-Pox should almost universally appear in a mild and favourable manner, nor is it possible to explain the fact upon any medical principle'.[9]

By 1820, faced with the apparent miracle of cowpox inoculation, Gilbert Blane, FRS, Physician in Ordinary to the King, could only bow down with something approaching reverence:

One can hardly contemplate with sufficient astonishment the extraordinary fact that a morbid poison taken from a domestic animal should, when inserted into the human body, shield it against the assault of one of the most fatal and cruel maladies to which it is incident [...] so that what seems at first sight merely a sportive aberration from the usual course of things, has, by the wise dispensation of Providence, become subservient to the most beneficent purposes.[10]

Forty years later, in his *Vaccination Papers*, John Simon, tactfully excluding Providence from the discussion, commented:

It remains one of the most interesting and least explained facts in pathology, that the specific contagion or ferment of small-pox, so uncontrollable in its operations when it enters a man in the ordinary way of his breathing an infected atmosphere, becomes for the most part disarmed of its virulence when it is artificially introduced to the system through a puncture of the skin...[11]

Yet another forty years on the mystery was referred to and magisterially dismissed in the final report of the Royal Commission on Vaccination (1896):

The precise *modus operandi* by which a previous attack of a disease furnishes security against a subsequent attack by the same disease has not yet been elucidated. There can be no cause for astonishment, then, if we are unable to trace the steps by which vaccination exerts a protective influence, supposing the fact that it does to be established, nor is it essential that we should succeed in tracing them. Our inability to accomplish this does not seem to us to be the slightest reason for regarding with doubt the conclusions to which the facts lead us.[12]

The phenomenon continued to remain inexplicable until the complexities of the body's immune system began to be unravelled early in the twentieth century, but in the absence of any understanding or even a plausible explanation of the physiological process on which the whole moral justification for compulsory vaccination depended, the medical profession, with the wholehearted backing of the legislature, pressed on cheerfully and relentlessly, with results summarized years later by a former Director of the Public Health Authority: 'Smallpox vaccine has probably been followed by more complications and been responsible for more deaths than any other vaccine. The practice of vaccination was carried on for about a hundred years before the nature and causation of its attendant risks began to be appreciated.'[13]

Seen against this perspective the objections and fears of the anti-vaccinationists appear somewhat less irrational than they were portrayed by the advocates of ruthless compulsion, and without going to the unfettered extremes of Creighton (and, as will appear, White) they had some justification for regarding Jenner, and before him Lady Mary Wortley Montagu, as the prime architects of their supposed misfortunes.

One of White's most vigorous and repeated assaults on Jenner had its origin in Jenner's candid and injudicious admission of the somewhat flimsy quality of the investigation on which he had based his theory of the relationship between horse grease and smallpox: 'although I have not been able to prove it from actual experiments conducted immediately under my own eye, yet the evidence I have adduced appears sufficient to establish it'.[14]

This was an astonishing assumption, and White made great play with it. 'Evidence adduced! Of evidence there was none. The farmers might be right in their opinion that Cow-pox sprang from Horse-Grease, but opinion was not evidence...'[15] As to Jenner's alleged thirty years' study of the subject:

> Until 1796 when he operated on Phipps he never made an experiment in Horse Grease Cow-pox Inoculation, and not until 1798, a few weeks before going to press with the *Inquiry* did he repeat the experiment; and though his later cases were complicated with erysipelas [...] he got together his scratch lot of cases [...] and consigned the concern, crude and incomplete, to the public.[16]

Horse grease, to mix a few metaphors, was Jenner's Achilles heel, and got him off on entirely the wrong foot. The relationship between smallpox, cowpox, horsepox and horse grease is a complex one and was the source of bitter controversy throughout much of the century and later. Were they the same disease, aspects of a common disease, totally unrelated? The problem has been unravelled by Derrick Baxby in his study *Jenner's Smallpox Vaccine* (1981) to which the reader is referred. The only point on which all parties soon came to agree was that horse grease had 'nothing to do with the case'; but the topic, quietly dropped from future publications by Jenner with, it was claimed, neither explanation nor apology, provided White with the refrain that he 'iterated' time and time again, in various forms, throughout his book:

'Let it suffice to say that the note of Jenner's *Inquiry* was Horse Grease Cowpox and nothing else. Strike at Horse Grease and the affair is reduced to nonentity.'[17]

A further source of contention was the distinction Jenner drew between 'true' and 'spurious' cowpox: what sort of disease, his enemies jeered, was 'spurious cowpox'? What he meant, and explained at length, was that there were various eruptions that appeared on the cow's teats that looked so similar to the casual eye that the farm workers would lump them all together under the general term 'cowpox', when only one kind of eruption produced 'true' cowpox matter, and even then only if it were transferred from its source to its intended recipient at a precise stage in its development. The explanation was logical enough to be convincing and had been accepted by most reputable observers in Jenner's own day, but the alleged confusion served as a useful weapon of ridicule against him for years to come.

Another source of criticism was that, having launched his theory on the medical world, Jenner had done so little to follow it up or attempt to validate it, as might have been expected of a conscientious researcher, so that it was left to others, notably Pearson and Woodville, to undertake the further investigation that was called for. Instead of settling himself in London, where he would have been at the centre of the medical establishment, able to defend himself against unscrupulous attacks, he spent most of his time in the village of Berkeley in Gloucestershire, where his home was, or in fashionable Cheltenham, where he had built up a lucrative practice. This reclusive lifestyle was dictated partly by concern for his wife's health, which remained a constant cause for anxiety, but Jenner was by temperament averse to city life, describing himself as a countryman, and 'cottagey'.

All this and a great deal more was eagerly seized on by White, enabling him to attack the image of the Great Benefactor with a litany of insults: Jenner had 'a loose and illogical mind' and 'essentially a mean spirit'; he was 'constitutionally deficient in method and assiduity – idle and self-indulgent', 'a quack, malicious, impudent', 'slippery', 'timid and indolent', 'a trumpery collector of gossip'. The measure of his claims was 'to define the truth there was in a popular belief, not to make an independent discovery'.

The remainder of White's attack on Jenner and vaccination consisted essentially of the usual barrages of statistics, together with claims that smallpox (a) was not as serious a disease as it was made out to be, and (b) was in any case on the decline from at least the time when Jenner was introducing the concept of vaccination as a prophylactic; but above all, that in the context of a parent's rights and responsibilities with regard to a child's health, compulsion imposed by the state was totally unacceptable on both moral and religious grounds:

> It is not in human nature to submit to the indignity of imposture: and to thousands of Englishmen vaccination is a cruel and degrading imposture, and to punish them for their loyalty to what they think right is every whit as tyrannical as it was for Catholics to persecute Protestants, and Protestants Catholics, and Catholics and Protestants [to persecute] Jews. There is no difference in the terms of intolerance and there is no difference in the spirit with which this latter day tyranny is confronted and that with which religious liberty was vindicated and won.[18]

The passions aroused by Jenner have inevitably subsided but he remains to some extent an ambiguous figure. To Dixon, writing in 1962, he was 'an inherently lazy man [...] a dreamer who, having made a rather lucky discovery, wanted to retire and continue to dream about natural history and its relation to disease in man'.[19] To Baxby in 1979, although Jenner's practical experience of vaccination was limited, he showed 'that the vaccine could be carried in series by arm-to-arm passage and [...] brought public attention to focus on the procedure [...] He deserves credit for appreciating the importance of vaccination'.[20]

There was one anti-vaccinationist who is better known than all the others put together, chiefly because of his renown in the much wider fields of drama, politics and general polemic. His most famous attack on vaccination was written when compulsion was virtually on its way out, but it is worth a comment because so many readers and play-goers, dazzled by his customary sweeping assumptions of omniscience, may be led into simply taking it at its highly misleading face value.

George Bernard Shaw, born in Dublin in 1856, was allegedly successfully vaccinated as one of the earliest children on whom the operation was performed in accordance with the recent Act of Parliament (the whole of Ireland being at the time part of the United Kingdom). There seems to be no evidence that he was ever revaccinated, a precaution strongly advocated when it became accepted that the protection afforded by primary vaccination was likely to have faded by the time a child reached the age of ten, or, as some authorities insisted, as young as three. In his mid-twenties, having transferred himself to London to try to earn a living as a writer, Shaw caught smallpox and according to his biographer, Michael Holroyd, emerged from the experience, which had deeply distressed him, as a confirmed anti-vaccinationist: 'Having studied the literature and statistics of smallpox he concluded that the case for fortifying the blood against the disease was unproven.'[21] At this period the tide of anti-vaccination literature was in full flood, and it is possible that Shaw may have been acquainted with some of the leaders of the opposition to the compulsory Act. As a vestryman in one of London's poorest parishes, St Pancras, he would also have had plenty of opportunities to observe the operation of the Act in practice (although it was never his lot to find himself among the ranks of dissenting parents). On at least one occasion, in 1902, in a letter to *The Times*, he made some rather wild accusations against the authorities and was challenged to substantiate them by the *British Medical Journal*. His riposte was largely a piece of bluster, which provoked a further onslaught from the *BMJ*, and he appears to have withdrawn from the contest.

Shaw's most outspoken and considered attack on vaccination was made in 1906. The occasion was the appearance of his play *The Doctor's Dilemma*, or more accurately the *Preface on Doctors* that accompanies it. In the course of the play one character says that he doesn't believe in morality: he's a disciple of Bernard Shaw; to which another character replies, 'Say no more, please. When a man pretends to discuss science, morals and religion and then avows himself a follower of a notorious and avowed anti-vaccinationist there is nothing more to be said.' The point of this Shavian jest a century on probably passes most audiences by (assuming that it hasn't been cut anyway).

A more memorable line in the play asserts that 'all professions are a conspiracy against the laity', which in this context means the medical profession. The fashionable Mayfair consultants in the cast, with their talk of 'nuciform sacs' and 'stimulating the phagocytes', are simply buffoons. A significant figure is the impoverished Doctor Blenkinsop, once a member of the élite himself, but now 'flabby and shabby, cheaply fed and cheaply clothed'. Doctors, the *Preface* asserts, are hideously poor. 'Better be a railway porter than an ordinary English medical practitioner.' They are also, in Shaw's view, charlatans. People imagined that the controversy concerning vaccination was a scientific one, when in fact it had nothing to do with science:

The medical profession, consisting for the most part of very poor men struggling to keep up appearances beyond their means, find themselves threatened with the extinction of a considerable part of their incomes: a part, too, that is easily and regularly earned, since it is independent of disease, and brings every person born into the nation, healthy or not, to the doctors [...] Under such circumstances, vaccination would be defended desperately were it twice as dirty, dangerous and unscientific as it actually is.[22]

White had held back from such a slander: 'Of course it would be absurd to charge medical men individually with defending vaccination because of the gain attached thereto [...] nothing of the kind is intended'.

Shaw's contempt for the medical profession extended far beyond the topic of vaccination. The evidence suggests that he was an adherent of the 'filth' explanation of the origin of disease. Taking one side in a controversy going back many years he rejected the concept of germs, denounced bacteriology as a 'superstition', and declared that the simplest way to kill most microbes is to throw them into an open street or river and let the sun shine on them. He ridiculed the notion of infection: he could remember, he said, when doctors no more dreamt of consumption and pneumonia being infections than 'so great and clinical observer as Sydenham' dreamt of smallpox being infectious. This casual reference to the seventeenth-century physician, of whom most of his readers were unlikely to have heard, must have seemed a telling stroke – Shaw at his most omniscient. It is amusing to be reminded by a modern authority on Sydenham of *obiter dicta* that strikingly anticipate the Shavian brand of witticism, as for example: 'anatomy, botany [...] nonsense, Sir! I know an old woman in Covent Garden who understands botany better, and as for anatomy, my butcher can dissect a joint full as well'. Another young hopeful, Richard Blackmore, asking Sydenham what books he should study in preparation for practising medicine, was told to go away and read *Don Quixote*.

Holroyd's assertion that Shaw had 'studied the literature of smallpox' is hardly borne out by the *Preface* to *The Doctor's Dilemma*, in which he makes at least two astonishing statements: 'Neither Jenner nor any other doctor ever, as far as I know, inculcated the popular notion that everybody got smallpox as a matter of course before vaccination was invented.' The only answer to this is a selective roll-call of witnesses, beginning with Rhazes, the tenth-century Arabian physician: 'Children, especially male, rarely escape being seized by this disease'. Then there is Shaw's much-admired Sydenham: 'The Small Pox of all other diseases is the most common, as that which, sooner or later (at least in this part of the world) attaques most men'. In 1736 Sir Hans Sloane, physician to King George the Second, President of both the Royal Society and the Royal College of Physicians, wrote that 'scarce one in a thousand misses having [smallpox] some time in their life'. Forty years later we find Mr Richard Brooke writing to James Pearson, Foreign Corresponding Secretary of the Royal Society, 'there are very few who escape having the smallpox sooner or later in life'. Baron Dimsdale, author of the standard late eighteenth-century textbook on the treatment of the disease, described it as 'a poison, the operation of which most of the human population are liable to experience once in their lives'.[23] Haygarth, the physician who studied the incidence of smallpox in Chester, wrote: 'The small-pox [...] has long been regarded as one of the necessary evils of humanity'.[24] Thomas Pruen noted in 1807 that although there had in the past been certain country districts where great numbers passed through life without ever having smallpox, 'now [...] from the extended communication between the most distant parts of the kingdom, an adult who has not undergone the small-pox is hardly to be found'.

These authorities, picked out more or less at random, bring us down to the early era of vaccination, Shaw's *terminus ad quem*. There is admittedly something a little suspicious in the repetition from generation to generation of a generalization perpetuated by a profession with a possible axe to grind, and Shaw would have been justified in expressing some degree of scepticism, but scepticism or doubt of any kind formed no part of his make-up. It may be that he had never come across these and similar sources, in which case his reading was less wide than is claimed for it; or he may have known of them but simply decided to ignore them as spoiling a good argument.

Even more astonishing is the second of his categorical statements, that 'it was really the public, and not the medical profession, that took up vaccination with irresistible faith, sweeping the invention out of Jenner's hands and establishing it in a form which he himself repudiated'. Jenner's *Inquiry* appeared in 1798. In 1802, four years later, 173 members of the London Medical Society, including many of the leading lights of the profession, published their testimonial regretting the 'unjust prejudice' that prevented the poor from 'laying hold of the advantages of the Cow-Pox', and making known their own opinion that 'the persons who have had the Cow-Pox are perfectly secure from the future infection of the Small-Pox'. How, White asked, did it ever come to pass that 'so many doctors signed the testimonial [...] when they had not and could not have, any experience to warrant their assertion?'[25] And why, he might have added, did Jenner spend so much time and ink lamenting that his own fellow-countrymen, almost alone in the civilized world, greeted with such indifference, not to say repugnance, the great blessing he had conferred on them?

CHAPTER 16

TEN SHILLINGS OR SEVEN DAYS

By 1906, when Shaw published his heterodox version of events, much of the steam had gone out of the vaccination controversy, as will be described in the proper place. In the heyday of White, Garth Wilkinson and others, who were caught up in it emotionally and in the law courts, it was still a burning issue. A hitherto slowly gathering movement of resentment erupted finally into open conflict with, at its heart, the 'cat-and-mouse' persecution of anti-vaccinationists that even Simon's biographer found difficult to excuse.

The effective starting point was the little-noticed Act of 1861, which empowered but did not specifically require boards of guardians to prosecute parents who neglected or refused to have a child vaccinated. In 1863 a Member of Parliament asked for a return of the number of unions and single parishes in England and Wales 'of which the guardians and overseers have taken measures to enforce obedience to the Vaccination Acts'. Figures produced by the Poor Law Board, in response to the question 'Whether measures have been taken', revealed the almost total failure of the Acts to achieve their professed aim:

Yes	(England)	77
Yes	(Wales)	7
No	(England)	424
No	(Wales)	34

Some boards had done 'nothing, beyond publishing notices, handbills, etc.' to remind parents of their duty. A small number had appointed someone – the clerk of the board or the local registrar – to enforce the law, but there was no evidence that a start had been made. Others were anxious to point to good intentions, but with no tangible progress to report: 'No, but subject to consideration'; 'No [but] have threatened proceedings'; 'No actual prosecutions taken'; 'No, but guardians intend to'; 'No, beyond refusing out-relief to parents whose children have not been vaccinated'. In eleven counties no action at all had been taken; two of them had not even bothered to issue the statutory notice to parents of newborn children. This was the position throughout the country when Simon's inspectors were engaged in their nationwide investigation into the quantity and quality of vaccination. The unavoidable conclusion was that enforcement of the law was something that boards of guardians did not want to become entangled in, especially if the costs of prosecutions were to be borne to any extent by the ratepayers.

The Act of 1867 tightened the law drastically, but still failed to provide the machinery indispensable to secure compliance. In 1870 a questioner asked in the Commons, with respect to the metropolitan district of London, how many vaccinations had been effected by public vaccinators as compared with the number of births registered. The answer was: registered births 112,250; vaccinations 41,404; successful vaccinations 40,842. In other words, of the children registered (almost certainly fewer than the number born) more than two thirds had not been vaccinated. Even allowing for the vast size of London, its constantly shifting population of often untraceable slum-dwellers and the number of children who did not survive long enough to become candidates for the vaccinator's lancet, the statistics pointed once again to the general and disastrous failure of the system.

The situation changed significantly with the appointment under the Act of 1871 of vaccination officers charged specifically with securing compliance with the Act. When the new arrangements had been given time to take effect a Member of Parliament asked for the number of prosecutions that had taken place in England and Wales between 1 January 1870 and 1 January 1875, distinguishing between those taken under section 29 of the 1867 Act and those under section 31. As a further refinement the questioner wished to be informed of the penalty imposed; whether the accused was imprisoned; if discharged, on what grounds. The results, tabulated county by county and town by town, incorporate too much detail to be more than roughly summarized, but show clearly how the justices of England and Wales had responded to the freedom and opportunities granted to them by the legislators and the judiciary.

Under section 29 there had been 1,394 prosecutions; under section 31, 342. Thirty defendants had been imprisoned under section 29, seven under section 31. Fines varied between 6*d*. and £1, costs, usually awarded, between 10 and 20*s*. The deterrent effect of a threat of prosecution was illustrated in a number of localities. In Dewsbury, a notoriously anti-vaccinationist town, 69 summonses were issued in 1870, of which 27 resulted in fines; the figures for 1871 were 96 summonses and a further 27 convictions. The remaining 111 summonses were withdrawn, presumably because in most cases the desired response, vaccination of the child, had been achieved. The long-standing drawback to compulsory legislation seemed at last to have been removed, but a severe and wholly unexpected reverse lay in wait for the authorities. The moment when the ring-fence of compulsory vaccination was finally riveted into place coincided with the arrival of what proved to be one of the worst disasters in the modern history of smallpox, the great pandemic of 1871–74.[1] In 1871, from the previous year's figure of just over 2,600, the number of deaths in England and Wales leapt to 23,062, with a further 19,022 in 1872, a total of 42,000, the majority according to Creighton, consisting of 'young persons and adults'.

The origin and exceptional gravity of the pandemic, which struck in almost every country in the world, were the subject of much debate. As far as Europe was concerned one of the chief contributory causes was held to be the Franco–Prussian war, which broke out in July 1870. The German army was well protected by vaccination and revaccination; the French army and the population in general were not. French prisoners of war, distributed among several countries, with a large contingent in Britain, were accused of having brought with them a particularly viru-lent and unfamiliar strain of smallpox.

Seaton, in his report of 1874 to the Local Government Board, admitted 'What was the mysterious "epidemic influence" which caused such peculiar intensity of the disease [...] is quite unknown to us', asserting at the same time that the epidemic had provided 'the complete answer [...] to the notion which of late had been ventilated by some, that small-pox is a disease tending naturally to extinction'. He further embarked on a lengthy exposition of the extent to which, he claimed, vaccination had protected the population, concluding that, '[i]t does not admit of reasonable doubt that the 16,812 smallpox deaths arising from the epidemic in England between the ages of 1 and 15 were, with comparatively few exceptions, the result of sheer neglect of vaccination', or, in a later passage, 'vaccination inefficiently performed', that is, during the period between the Acts of 1853 and 1867.

As might be expected, anti-vaccinationists took the opposite view, arguing that the epidemic proved that the protection that vaccination was alleged to provide was, as they had always insisted, an illusion. The years following the epidemic in England and Wales gave ammunition to both sides. Epidemics in particular locations pushed the annual figure of deaths as high as 4,278 in 1877, whereas in 1890 the nation-wide total was a mere 16 in a population that had increased during the interval.

Meanwhile, as recent legislation brought more and more defaulters and objectors within the reach of the law, the campaign against them was stepped up. The rigour of magistrates varied from area to area: seven prosecutions in Dorset (a very sparsely populated county), 105 in Gloucester, 168 in Lancaster, 220 in Durham. The 'cat-and-mouse' effect is also discernible: two or three prosecutions in respect of the same child were not uncommon, and examples occur that imply persecution on a grand scale. In Hertford there were only six prosecutions under section 29 but 59 under section 31, of which 19 were suffered by an offender referred to only as 'J.P.', and a further 12 by 'H.S.' The unfortunate 'J.P.' paid a total of £14 at least in fines, a very considerable sum a century ago. Imprisonment, as the totals show, was less common at this stage, but when resorted to was relatively severe. In Chesterfield, out of 27 prosecutions under section 31, two resulted in sentences of seven days, and nine of 14 days.

Prosecutions were sometimes so brutal that even supporters of compulsion were moved to protest. Under the heading 'How to make Vaccination Unpopular' (17 June 1871), the *Lancet* reported a particularly vicious example:

> The authorities of Islington [...] summoned a poor man named Jones for not taking his children to the vaccination station to have their arms inspected. The man, who appeared very ill, and who had risen from his bed to obey the summons, stated that he had been told by the district medical officer not to take the children to the station because there was small-pox in the house, and a child still lying dead in the next room, and it seemed to both that there was a danger of spreading the disease in this way. The magistrate nevertheless fined the man 20 shillings on each summons, or in default 14 days' imprisonment in the House of Correction. The defendant, who had not a farthing of money, was removed in a prison van...[2]

The *Lancet* commented, 'It seems to us that this man has been most cruelly treated. So far from being forced to take his children to the public station, to propagate small-pox among unprotected children [who were waiting to be vaccinated] there ought to be a law forbidding the use of public stations by anyone residing in an infected house'.

Another victim of the Vaccination Act was Charles Washington Nye, a Chatham man, whose case first gained notoriety when it was brought to the attention of the select committee in 1871.[3] His tribulations began in 1868, when he was imprisoned in Canterbury gaol for 14 days for not having had one of his children vaccinated. 'At the end of my sentence I was turned adrift to go to Chatham, twenty-eight miles, in the best way I could without a farthing in my pocket.' After he had made further appearances in court the chairman of the board of guardians wanted no more charges to be brought, but his colleagues thought otherwise and several prosecutions followed. In the course of 1870 Nye served a sentence of 14 days in March, 31 days in July and 31 days in December, during which periods his wife and children had to go into the workhouse. He himself was employed in pushing loaded wheelbarrows at the foundations of a new cookhouse:

> I worked at that until my hands got so bad that the handles of every barrow I wheeled were stained with my blood, and I refused to work at it any longer. I was then put on the task of oakum-picking, and after I had been supplied with my supper gruel a warder came and took it away, remarking that as I was too lazy to work I was not entitled to it.

In 1872 he served a sentence of 31 days in Maidstone gaol. It was not until the mid-1890s that the Royal Commission on Vaccination succeeded, against strong opposition, in securing more humane treatment for jailed opponents of compulsion.

As time passed there were signs of confusion as to what degree of compulsion it was legitimate to apply. In 1876 the guardians of the Evesham union enquired of the Local Government Board, with reference to a parent who had refused to have his child vaccinated, whether they had 'discretionary powers' to abstain from taking any further legal proceedings against persons who had been fined more than once for this offence. Their bewilderment was understandable in view of the passing in 1874 of an Act that gave the Local Government Board the power to override a decision by guardians not to carry out a prosecution. The reply, from the President of the LGB, George Sclater-Booth, was a classic of its kind:

> It is distinctly contemplated by Article 16 of the Board's General Order of 31st October 1874 that, independently of any proceedings which may be taken against the person in default under section 29 of the Vaccination Act of 1867, the vaccination officer

shall be authorized to take proceedings against him if he continue contumacious at least once under section 31.[4]

Until this procedure had been followed and a conviction obtained, the Board considered that 'the several means which the law provides with a view to ensure the vaccination of a child have not been used'; and by implication should be used. However, the vaccination officer must not prosecute more than once under section 31 'without the express instructions of the guardians'. So where did that leave the guardians? They should 'carefully consider' what effect a continuance of proceedings would be likely to have 'in procuring the vaccination of the individual child and in insuring the observance of the law in the Union generally'. And what considerations might be allowed to influence their decision? It was, on the one hand, undeniable that 'a repetition of legal proceedings' had sometimes resulted in the vaccination of a child when previous prosecutions had failed: but, on the other hand, the Board was prepared to admit that when in a particular case repeated prosecutions had failed in their object 'it becomes necessary to carefully consider the question whether the continuance of a fruitless contest with the parent may not have a tendency to produce mischievous results, by exciting sympathy with the person prosecuted, and thus creating a more extended opposition to the law'. This of course was the argument that had prompted the addition to the Act of 1871 of the clause that Lord Redesdale had so successfully demolished.

So once again, where did this leave the guardians? The law appeared to be unequivocal – they had a duty to secure the vaccination of the child; but their masters at the Poor Law Board 'entertain no doubt that [the guardians] will not fail to exercise the *discretionary powers* [author's italics] confided to them in the manner best calculated to give effect to the policy of the law'. This masterpiece of equivocation, or common sense, according to how it was interpreted, was ordered to be printed and was distributed to all boards of guardians.

As the 1880s approached the tempo of the campaign against defaulters accelerated. A parliamentary return dated 1879 showed that the total number of fines imposed had risen to 3,929. Seventy-three offenders had been imprisoned for 14 days or less, 14 others for periods up to one month. These figures were admitted to be an understatement. Some districts had made no return for part of the period, and the returns from others related to the number of persons prosecuted, rather than to the number of prosecutions.

* * *

During these years the anti-vaccinationists had not been inactive. It was the period of the *Vaccination Tracts*, and a reorganization and strengthening of the movement. After the well-meant but somewhat amateurish efforts of the early agitators, typified by Pitman in Manchester, the task of organizing resistance to the Vaccination Acts was taken over by more seasoned and sophisticated campaigners and social reformers in London and the south. Not all of them were free of some taint of crankiness, and others, often loosely summed up as 'radicals', were conspicuous for their support for any cause which might be described as 'anti'.

The first Anti-Compulsory Vaccination League had been set up in London in response to the 1867 Act, and a number of towns and cities, mostly in the north, had soon followed suit. There was little in the way of organization, the numbers of protesters were unknown, and the press in general showed considerable unwillingness to lend support to what was mostly seen as an unpopular cause.

The Act of 1874, which increased the powers of the Local Government Board over boards of guardians, stirred the anti-vaccinationists to further efforts. The Hume-Rotherys, now living in Cheltenham, founded a National Anti-Compulsory Vaccination League, which was less successful on the national scale than had been hoped for owing to the inability of the northern leagues to offer much by way of financial contributions, which in turn reduced the effectiveness of the parent body. Nevertheless, the following year produced one of the outstanding engagements so far in the anti-vaccination struggle.

The location was the town of Keighley in what was then the West Riding of Yorkshire where, in contrast to developments elsewhere in the country, the local board of guardians, with clear public backing and relying on the discretion apparently allowed them by the Evesham letter, dropped all prosecutions of parents and sacked their vaccination officer.[5] The Local Government Board felt it could not overlook insubordination on this scale and intervened to restore the status quo, but after several skirmishes, which ended with seven of the Keighley guardians being briefly incarcerated in York Castle, the Board retreated in disorder and released the men. In MacLeod's words, the Board was

> caught in a series of contradictions: it had exerted legal but unwise authority over local functionaries in a questionable manner; it had inadequately assessed the position of the Guardians and the nature of local opposition; it had summarily enforced central policy upon local administration after urging the Guardians to use discretion; it had imprisoned men who were among the

leaders of their community; and it had almost made state medicine an enemy of the people.[6]

To the anti-vaccinationists the outcome was a famous victory. An outburst of confused rhetoric from the Hume-Rotherys ended with a clarion call: 'Three cheers for Keighley and the seven champions! And may God defend the right!' But one victory does not necessarily terminate a war, and this conflict had the better part of a generation to run before the obduracy of the party of compulsion could be finally made to crumble. The anti-vaccinationists had gained publicity and enthused their own supporters in particular localities, but at the expense of appearing to be extremists deliberately seeking martyrdom, as more than one embittered opponent from the medical profession complained. On the wider front they had neither drummed up mass support for their stand nor, more importantly, won over a significant number of Members of Parliament, without whose active goodwill the hated compulsory law could not be repealed. For this purpose something more impressive and better organized was needed than spasmodic guerrilla warfare in small provincial towns. The outcome was the formation of yet another pressure group, the London Society for the Abolition of Compulsory Vaccination. Launched in 1880 it numbered among its leaders William White as secretary and William Tebb, a Manchester man who was both an FRGS and an FZS, with a long experience of promoting sanitary reform. The long-term aim of the Society was the total repeal of the Vaccination Acts, possibly as the result of a Royal Commission appointed to look into the whole subject of vaccination.

The achievement of even this first step was still more than a decade away, but the zeal and professionalism of the new Society transformed the situation. With wealthy backing, the promotion of educational programmes, public lectures, conferences, its own offices in London and its own monthly journal, *The Vaccination Inquirer*, the Society began to build up a strong membership throughout the country, with links to sympathetic organizations in other countries.

In the meantime, with no restraint on their activities beyond the tentative suggestions made in the Evesham letter, boards of guardians, backed by willing magistrates, had tended to make the most of the powers at their disposal. An outstanding example was to be found in the city of Leicester, which had long been known for its radical and non-conformist temper in respect of a number of issues. One of the earliest Anti-Vaccination Leagues in the country was formed there in 1869, and the first jail sentence for a breach of the Vaccination Act was passed on a Leicester man. The city was poised for a stand-off between the political and medical establishments and the power of local anti-establishment feeling.

As a result of the large number of deaths from smallpox that occurred during the great pandemic of the early 1870s the local authority had insisted on the Vaccination Acts being applied with exceptional rigour. As the panic died down so did the zeal of the city's health department, but not that of some of the boards of guardians. By October 1884, according to MacLeod, 966 cases of default had been prosecuted and 23 fathers sent to jail. The justice system could not cope with the growing pressure, and a year later there were said to be more than 4,000 people awaiting summonses. An anonymous letter in the staunchly anti-vaccinationist *Leicester Mercury* conveyed the atmosphere in the city:

> Much has been said at different times lately about the action the magistrates take when cases are brought before them in which people, from conscientious motives, and anxious to do their best for their children, are fined for not having their little ones vaccinated. The Leicester bench say they are only administering the law, and that there is no other course open; 'ten shillings or 7 days' are now so well-known as to be bywords in Leicester. Whilst some anxious parent is describing the suffering or even the death of a little one from vaccination, as a cause why another should not be vaccinated, you may see the bench not listening, but in earnest conversation on some other topic, only pausing to say '10 shillings or 7 days'.[7]

The pages of the *Mercury* carried a steady stream of evidence in support of the reader's complaint, by contrast with the *Courier* which virtually ignored the subject:

> George Banford had a child born in 1868. It was vaccinated and after the operation the child was covered with sores, and it was some considerable time before it was able to leave the house. Again Mr. Banford complied with the law in 1870. This child was vaccinated by Dr. Sloane in the belief that by going to him they would get purer matter. In that case erysipelas set in, and the child was on a bed of sickness for some time. In the third case the child was born in 1872 and soon after vaccination erysipelas set in and it took such a bad course that at the expiration of 14 days the child died.[8]

Being unwilling to put a fourth child at risk Mr Banford was fined ten shillings with the option of seven days in prison. The choice he made was not reported.

Another offender seems to have fallen foul of the notorious section 31 of the Act:

> Melton Mowbray Petty Sessions. Edward Irons was summoned for neglecting to comply with an order for the vaccination of his son, aged two years. He said he had a conscientious objection to conforming to the Vaccination Act, and he was also acting under the advice of his doctor, who stated that vaccination was not conducive to the child's health, nor would it benefit him. One of his children had been vaccinated, and she had suffered considerably from the effects of it, and he could not allow the boy to undertake the same risk. He then gave the opinions of several medical gentlemen on the evils of vaccination, and said he thought it would be inadvisable for the Bench to enforce the law upon a conscientious objection. The Chairman said there were few questions which had given rise to more varied opinions than the subject of vaccination. It had been proved beyond doubt that vaccination had caused smallpox to show itself in a much milder form. The Bench were unanimous in their opinions upon the question. They acted upon public grounds, and decided that the order should be enforced within a fortnight. If the order were not complied with, defendant would be liable to a penalty of twenty shillings. That course would be taken with all cases that came before them.[9]

The state of public opinion was demonstrated by the scene that greeted the decision of a small band of objectors who had chosen the more severe of the alternatives offered by the justices:

> By about 7.30 a goodly number of anti-vaccinators were present, and an escort was formed preceded by a banner, to accompany a young mother and two men, all of whom had resolved to give themselves up to the police and undergo imprisonment in preference to having their children vaccinated. The utmost sympathy was expressed to the poor woman, who bore up bravely, and although seeming to feel her position expressed her determination to go to prison again and again rather than give her child over to the 'tender mercies' of a public vaccinator. The three were attended by a numerous crowd and in Gallowtreegate three hearty cheers were given for them, which were renewed with increased vigour as they entered the doors of the prison cells.[10]

The harshest penalty of all, where the poor were concerned, followed when magistrates decided to invoke the law governing the non-payment of debt:

> A man named Arthur Ward had two children injured through vaccination and refused to submit another one to the operation. A fine was imposed and on 24th November two police officers called for the penalty, or in default to ticket the goods. The husband was out at the market, and the poor woman had no money to pay. The goods downstairs were considered insufficient to cover the amount, and the officers demanded to go upstairs. The woman refused to allow this, and an altercation took place, and harsh language was used by the officers, who threatened to take her husband to prison, terrifying Mrs. Ward. At that time she was pregnant, and the shock to the system, and the fright were of such a character that symptoms ensued which ultimately led to a premature confinement, and on 26th December she gave birth to a still-born child. She never recovered and last week she expired. The doctor who had attended Mrs. Ward said that although he believed in vaccination he did not think it was the duty of any professional man to carry out the laws in the outrageous and brutal manner in which they were enforced.[11]

The state of feeling in the city did not go unnoticed by the London Society, which decided to turn it to advantage. A mass protest against the compulsory Acts, centred on Leicester, was organized in March 1885. Contingents of supporters numbering more than 20,000 from more than 50 towns and cities throughout the British Isles gathered to listen to speeches from leaders of the movement and to march through the streets with a great parade of banners and dramatic tableaux. Full accounts appeared in the *Vaccination Inquirer*, the *Leicester Mercury* and numerous other papers. Typical of the tableaux was one that repre-sented

> a skeleton vaccinating an infant in its mother's lap while a policeman grips her uplifted hand, the mother's face being full of agony, while the skeleton and the officer of the law are grinning with horrid impressiveness. Other trollies contained 'furniture seized for blood-money', showing that [...] somebody was sleeping without a bedstead and sitting down to dinner, if he had one, without tables and chairs, instead of a baby being vaccinated. One trolley appeared to have negotiated the loan of the gallows from the

county gaol for Dr. Jenner's sole and particular use, and the execution was carried out without the slightest hitch, about every thirty yards, through some miles of streets amid strong manifestations of popular approval.[12]

Among dozens of banners and slogans one seemed to sum up the spirit and purpose of the demonstration:

From horse grease, calf-lymph, cowpox and the Local Government Board, good Lord deliver us!

Government sources were constantly at pains to issue assurances that 'the number of cases in which non-vaccination was due to direct refusal on the part of parents to comply with the law [...] constitutes an insignificant proportion of cases', but as events in Leicester showed the true measure of opposition to the law was not the number of parents punished but the amount of support they received among the population as a whole, which included many who might have joined the ranks of 'martyrs' if the probable consequences for them had not been too alarming to contemplate.

CHAPTER 17

DEATH BY NON-VACCINATION

Following the mass demonstration the Leicester guardians voted by 26 to eight to cease prosecutions. There was no response from the Local Government Board, but a carefully worded passage in a report by its Medical Officer of Health, written before the demonstration took place, illustrated clearly the Board's awareness of the dilemma with which the advocate of compulsion was confronted:

> Whether or not, in face of the accumulated evidence of the importance of vaccination to children, who cannot judge for themselves of its value, it may be expedient to relax those provisions of the Compulsory Vaccination Acts which allow of repeated penalties on such parents as refuse vaccination, is a question which lies within the province of the statesman rather than the physician to settle. To the physician, who realises the powers of vaccination, and who knows the malignity of the disease against which it protects, the notion of enforcing the acceptance of such a boon is distressful. But the distress is akin to that with which he himself has at times to force nourishment down the throat of a lunatic who is starving himself; and in the case of vaccination he sees that it is for the security of children otherwise helpless, not the recalcitrant himself, that compulsion is wanted.
>
> In England, however, 'compulsory vaccination' has never meant, and probably never will mean, taking a child out of the custody of its parent and returning it to him vaccinated; and if it does not mean this it may by some persons be judged advantageous, in order to avoid gratifying the sheer love of martyrdom that influences the conduct of misguided people, to alter the Compulsory Vaccination Acts in such a way as to limit the number of penalties that can be imposed for disobedience to them. I express no opinion on this proposal, but if it should be adopted it would appear as a

corollary that the Acts be so further altered as to mark by law the sense of the community that a parent will have committed an offence whose child dies of small-pox without having been vaccinated [...] Such parents will have failed to give the security that the law provides for their helpless children, and will be in the same position as if they had failed to provide their children with any other security important to their lives.[1]

This veiled attempt to broaden the nature of the offence committed by a defaulting parent was nothing new. As far back as 1856 the Bill with which Simon had hoped to launch his revision of the Vaccination Act had included a clause that showed the way things might be going:

In the case of the death from small-pox of any child born since the twelfth of August 1853 it shall be lawful for the coroner having jurisdiction in the sub-district, on receipt of notice [...] to summon a jury for the holding of an inquest of the body of such child...

If it were proved that the child had not been vaccinated,

the jury shall find accordingly and the coroner shall notify such verdict to the guardians or overseer [...] who may thereupon proceed against [the] parent [...] for the recovery of the penalty imposed by the Act.

The clause was lost with the withdrawal of the Bill and not restored in any subsequent legislation, but as time went by some coroners began to take the hint and hold inquests on unvaccinated children. This inevitably aroused fury among anti-vaccinationists and raised unanswered questions concerning the legality and intended purpose of an inquest.

An early reference, dating from the end of the twelfth century, indicated that the coroner's function was to inquire into 'unnatural' or unexplained deaths. Blackstone later defined the court of the coroner as 'a court of record to inquire, when anyone dies in prison or comes to a violent or sudden death, by what manner he came to his end'. The drawback to this concept, as William Farr pointed out in 1841, was that words such as 'violent', 'unnatural', 'sudden' were never defined, nor in fact were the conditions in which an inquest should be held explicitly stated.

The whole subject was clouded by so much uncertainty that in 1860 a select committee was appointed 'to consider the state of the law and practice as regards the taking of inquisitions in cases of death'. Among the issues identified by the committee in its report was a conflict of opinion between coroners and magistrates as to the circumstances in which an inquest should be held:

> The coroners contend that an inquest should be held in every case of violent or [...] 'unnatural death'; [...] on the other hand it is contended that no inquest should be held unless some suspicion exists that the death was caused by the wilful act of the deceased, or by some other person, or by negligence.[2]

The dispute centred on whether money was being wasted on unnecessary inquests, but the significant word from the point of view of the vaccination controversy was 'negligence', which was picked up in the Annual Report of the Registrar General for 1863:

> Smallpox exists now almost by sufferance, but owing to neglect, or to the inefficient practice of vaccination, 1,320 deaths by smallpox were registered.
>
> It is impossible to determine in these cases who is to blame in not procuring for the helpless children the protection which the law has provided against smallpox. The coroners, by holding a certain number of inquests, might ascertain how the matter really stands, and may prevent acts of negligence which in their consequences are as fatal as the ordinary offences of manslaughter.

This was clear enough but there was a further complication, resulting from the passage in 1836 of the Registration Act, which came to have a significant bearing on the position of defaulting parents. In the past, as Farr pointed out, 'juries did not ascertain "the cause of death" in several thousands of inquests'. Under the Act of 1836 a whole new duty was imposed on them: 'in any case in which an inquest shall be held upon any dead body the jury shall inquire of the particulars [...] required to be registered concerning the death and the coroner shall inform the registrar of the finding of the jury and the registrar shall make an entry accordingly'. Three years after the passing of the Act the Registrar General, in his first annual report 'earnestly recommended that every practising member of any branch of the medical profession who may have been present at the death, or in attendance during the last illness of any person' should give to anyone 'who may probably be required to give information, written statements of the cause of death which such persons may show to the Registrar and give as their information on the subject'.

This eased the new burden placed on jurors but only by adding to those of medical practitioners, who were advised that the statements required should be 'short and contain only the name of the disease considered to have been the cause of death, not a detailed account either of antecedent symptoms or appearances [...] after death'. The statement should 'exhibit' the popular or common name of the disease in preference to 'such as is known only to medical men'.

This again was clear enough in intention but the difficulty faced by medical men was that no precise or universally accepted terminology existed for their use when specifying in what manner the deceased had 'come to his end'. The common practice had been to fall back on popular but unhelpful phrases: 'putting on damp clothes', 'frozen to death', '*felo de se*', 'spontaneous combustion'. It was Farr who came to their rescue, removing the obstacle by issuing a 'Statistical Nosology to assist those who return causes of death'.[3] The terms listed were those recommended to be used in the first columns of registers; synonyms might be used in other columns 'at the discretion of the medical informant'.

Under the heading 'Epidemic, Endemic and Contagious Diseases' the following terms were permissible:

1(a) SMALL-POX (natural) with the alternative 'Variola'. 'Without previous vaccination of any kind' is to be always understood. The varieties of small-pox may be distinguished.

1(b) Small-pox (second attack)

1(c) Small-pox after Cow-pox. This entry is never to be used unless the vaccination have left a cicatrix – nor even until 30 days have elapsed after vaccination [...]

These precise definitions, worked out more than ten years before the passage of the first Act requiring compulsory vaccination, revealed their full significance in the years following the second and third Acts (1867, 1871) when anti-vaccinationists, less able to circumvent the law, were blaming vaccination for the deaths of their children. Coroners, relying on the Registrar General's hint of 1863, began a campaign against defaulting parents that, if logically carried through, could have placed them in greater jeopardy than they faced even under the Vaccination Acts.

One of the earliest to take the new line was Edwin Lankester, the coroner for West Middlesex, a former member of Simon's staff in the Medical Office of the Privy Council and, since 1856, Medical Officer of

Health of St James, a poor district of London. Described as 'robust', 'active and somewhat pugnacious', he took a great interest in sanitary reform. During a very severe epidemic of smallpox in London in 1867 he read a paper to the Social Sciences Association in the course of which he made his position clear:

> Feeling convinced that the neglect of vaccination is one of the great causes of the origin and spread of this foul disease I have felt it my duty to hold inquests in those cases which have come to my knowledge where children have died from this disease without being vaccinated. I have thought that the inquiry was within the spirit of the Coroner's Court, which inquires into the causes of all deaths that might have been prevented by proper and reasonable forethought and provision.[4]

The question had never been decided in a court of law but it was worth investigation,

> whether according to the spirit in which the verdict of manslaughter is returned in other cases, persons breaking the law in neglecting to have their children vaccinated are not exposed to a verdict of manslaughter, if it can be shown that [the children] have died from not having been vaccinated as the law requires.

The *Lancet*, wholly committed, like most of the medical profession, to compulsory vaccination, thought Lankester's stance 'worthy of approval', but the political establishment, engaged in putting the Vaccination Act of that year on the statute book, did not take the opportunity to add a charge of manslaughter to the threats already hanging over contumacious parents, and was in fact soon to be considering reducing the number of penalties to be inflicted on them.

A notorious inquest conducted by Lankester was investigated by the select committee of 1871. A doctor's certificate had given the cause of death of a recently vaccinated child as 'erysipelas'. The parent, Aaron Emery, objected, maintaining that the cause should be shown as 'vaccination'. Having overheard something suspicious at the inquest on another child he somewhat ill-advisedly asked Lankester to hold an inquest on his own son. Lankester agreed and the jury brought in a verdict of 'Died from erysipelas caused by vaccination'. Emery described for the committee what happened next:

> Dr. Lankester said, 'Gentlemen, you must modify this verdict and

put "misadventure" or "by accident"', and the foreman of the jury said he should do nothing of the kind: they had returned a verdict and they had done with it.[5]

Having confirmed in court that the verdict would be recorded as returned by the jury Emery let the matter rest, until a question arose as to the inscription to be placed on the child's tombstone. It was then discovered that without consulting anyone Lankester had rewritten the jury's verdict to read: 'William Emery was found dying and did die of the mortal effects of erysipelas, coming after vaccination, and the said jurors further say that the said death arose from misadventure', which was what the jurors had specifically declined to say. The committee was not told how the disagreement was resolved. Emery denied being an anti-vaccinationist, or having ever heard of an Anti-Vaccination League.

According to White, Lankester's defence was that 'vaccination was not a cause of death recognized by the law', by which he presumably meant Farr's *Nosology*. He died in 1874 and was succeeded in his office by a hardliner similar to himself. *Vaccination Tract No. 13* reported that 'coroner Hardwicke now holds inquests on unvaccinated children who died of small-pox, and the verdict makes non-vaccination itself into a violent death, the small-pox being left out of the record. DEATH BY NON-VACCINATION, a new spectre in nosology.'

* * *

By contrast with the happy-go-lucky approach to smallpox vaccination that had prevailed in the early days, specific and detailed instructions were issued to public vaccinators employed by contract under the terms of the compulsory Acts.[6] However, there was inevitably a great deal of slipshod workmanship in surgeries where the principles of sterilization and scrupulous cleanliness were little understood or, if inconvenient, disregarded.

The instructions, although modified and amplified from time to time, conformed to a standard pattern. Only children who were in good health should be vaccinated: 'do not vaccinate where there has been recent exposure to infection of measles or scarlatina' (the causes of many more deaths than smallpox), 'nor where erysipelas is prevailing in or about the place of residence [...] Direct care should be taken for keeping the vesicles' (the eruptions produced by vaccination) 'uninjured during their progress [...] Do not use any needless means of "protection" or of "dressing" to a vaccinated arm'. So much for recipients of lymph – the vaccinated. What of the donors – the 'vaccinifers', themselves of course by definition babies of less than three months old? 'Take lymph only from subjects who are in good health and as far as you can ascertain, of healthy parentage, preferring children whose families are known to you [...] Always carefully examine the subject as to any existing skin disease, and especially as to any signs of hereditary syphilis'.

The theory was clear enough, the practice often rather less so. Overcrowded urban stations; under-used stations in sparsely populated rural areas, where it was barely possible to maintain enough cases to keep up the arm-to-arm succession; hard-pressed working-class mothers trying to get through their daily tasks while reaching for any help in comforting babies with sore arms; vaccination officers trying to keep track of families moving every few weeks from one district to another in search of work, or 'flitting' from collectors of rent they couldn't pay; the downside of the vaccination service was always present, for the most part buried under self-congratulatory statistics, but surfacing occasionally in the form of tragedies too harrowing to be hushed up.

'Report to the Local Government Board by Mr J. Netten Radcliffe of certain cases of ERYSIPELAS following upon VACCINATION in the Misterton district of the Gainsborough Union, Lincolnshire'. Mr Radcliffe's report was published as a Return to an Order of the House of Commons.[7] Being a very full and scrupulous investigation it tends to obscure the essential facts, which were that of vaccinations carried out on 16 children by the public vaccinator, Dr Thomas Bell Wright, with lymph taken from the arm of a healthy child (who had himself been vaccinated with dried lymph supplied by the National Vaccine Establishment) four operations were unsuccessful – they did not 'take'; of the 12 that were 'more or less successful' ten children developed erysipelas, of whom six died.

The investigation was made difficult chiefly because the register of public vaccinations had not been kept properly, and Dr Wright 'has no record of the events [and] his memory is imperfect'. It was clear, however, that 'something in the mode of performing the vaccination had contributed to, if not actually determined, the subsequent erysipelas' and that 'the way in which the public vaccination had been carried out was altogether at variance with the instructions [given to] the public vaccinator'. In several aspects of his vaccinating the doctor was 'reprehensively careless'. The lancets he was accustomed to use were 'rusty and found to be dirty, both blades and handles'. Some points (ivory tips for use with reconstituted dried lymph) that he produced for examination 'can only be described as filthy'. These were the tools with which he opened the vesicles, or sores, on the arms of vaccinifers to transfer and insert lymph into the hitherto unblemished arms of the new arrivals.

The report included brief accounts of the accommodation in which some of the deceased children had been living:

Henderson: the cottage is wholly without drainage, and the ground immediately in front of the door was, at the time of the inquiry, saturated with slop water.

Baker: [...] the principal living room looks upon a small yard, surrounded by a high wall, in which are placed an earth closet, the ash bin and the water butt [...] The yard, in fact, forms a tank of comparatively stagnant air, liable at times to considerable fouling...

Smith: [...] adjoining the house is a stagnant ditch, reported to receive the drainage from a butcher's yard. The stench from this ditch was almost unendurable...

Smallpox was not a 'filth disease', and did not 'cause' erysipelas, but when it is recalled that children less than three months old were routinely being sent away from crowded vaccination stations with open wounds in their arms, to be tended in often vile conditions by parents ignorant through no fault of their own of the most elementary notions of hygiene or proper care in the case of illness, it is perhaps not to be wondered at that deaths occurred, and that conscientious and better-informed parents could be driven to protest against legislation compelling them to submit their children to surgery in conditions that no legislator or civil servant would have accepted for his own family.

Six years after the deaths in the Gainsborough area there was a similar tragedy in Norwich, where four children died of erysipelas and five were gravely ill in circumstances that pointed to 'something connected with vaccination', either on the day of the operation or, in two cases, on the day when the children were taken back for routine inspection. The vaccination station concerned was also the private residence of the vaccinator. One witness stated that the waiting room was crowded and occasionally some of the women and infants had to be accommodated in a private room upstairs.[8]

The conclusion reached by investigators of the outbreak of erysipelas was that it had been caused by 'some abnormal peculiarity or contamination of the lymph'. This did not satisfy the Medical Officer of Health of the Local Government Board, Dr Buchanan, who looked into the matter himself and passed a much more severe judgement on the public vaccinator for using the same ivory points for more than one operation. It was clear to him that 'in the sitting (on one of the days in question) a group of imperfectly cleaned points came into use' to transfer lymph, which would become infected during the process, to the arms of the children who had died or become ill. He proposed to issue a new instruction forbidding the practice.

The whole affair provided the occasion for outspoken criticism in a speech by Dr W. J. Collins, a university scholar and Member of the Royal College of Surgeons, at a meeting of the London Society for the Abolition of Compulsory Vaccination. Collins was a leading anti-vaccinationist but by no means one of the ranting emotional variety. 'We must not be too prone,' he said, 'to accept all evidence against vacci-nation without sifting it.'

The inspectors had said that pure lymph could not possibly do any harm, and had argued that 'because in such and such cases evil did result the lymph must have been impure'. They had entirely failed to see, Collins argued, that 'lymph, the impurity of which can only be tested by its results, is no better than lymph which is confessedly impure. When a child is dead of erysipelas it is too late to discover that the virus is impure'.[9] The vaccinator had admitted that he did not comply specifically with the instructions of the Board but, Collins asserted, 'it is sheer impossibility to carry these instructions out fully in the hurry and routine of a public vaccination station, and simply shows the utter impracticability and injustice of a system which it is perfectly impossible to adopt'.

Among Collins's own conclusions was that

in vaccination we use an animal poison whose mode of action is unknown to us, and whose effects we cannot measure; and that no amount of care and caution can obviate a repetition of disasters like that which has recently shocked us at Norwich. Such being the case it is the grossest tyranny to continue the compulsory enforcement of vaccination...[10]

If it came down to 'a balance of advantages, a choice of evils, an alter-native of risks, is it too much to ask that a parent should have the right to choose for himself and his child?'

CHAPTER 18

THE GREAT POX

If there was one source of danger that ranked above even erysipelas in the minds of anti-vaccinationists it was syphilis – the Great Pox, the 'disease of diseases'. The argument dated as far back as the years when Lady Mary Wortley Montagu was in the vanguard of advocates of the 'Byzantine Operation'. In one of the earlier adverse comments William Wagstaffe suggested in 1722 that an inoculator might seriously reflect

> that when he injects matter into the blood in this way it may be possible and even probable to communicate another Distemper, besides the Small Pox. Suppose the person the matter is taken from has the King's Evil, the Pox, Madness or some other inveterate disease. What would be the consequence of the method in such a case?

In the following year Sir Richard Blackmore, in a *Treatise upon the Small-Pox*, raised the same objection:

> it is very probable, that the seeds of other distempers may be communicated with those of the Small-Pox, contained in the prurient matter taken from the ripe pustules of the patient […] It is allowed that the principles of the King's Evil, of Consumption, Lunacy, and Venereal Disease are conveyed from fathers to their children successively through many generations: and are therefore called hereditary: a sad inheritance![1]

These warnings were not seriously taken up, perhaps because during the first twenty or so years from the introduction of inoculation the number of operations performed could be counted in hundreds, and the possibility that 'other distempers' could be 'insinuated' with the smallpox could be discounted. 'I know of no instance in so many years as this practice has subsisted where such accident has happened,' James Burges wrote in 1744, 'therefore I think it may be presumed that no such thing can happen, but that the matter of the small-pox is a poison *sui generis*, and can admit no other mixture'.[2] At the end of the century Daniel Sutton, who had practised his 'new' system of inoculation for thirty years, asserted that 'neither inveterate strumours, scrophulous complaints nor venereal taints (the most of all to be dreaded) have ever to my knowledge been communicated by the ordinary method of inoculation'.[3]

Even in the early days of vaccination when Jenner's enemies, chiefly Moseley, Rowley and 'Squirrel', the 'Anti-Vaccs' as he called them, were feeding the public alarming stories of the horrific effects of cowpox on the human body – the 'beastly breakings out of the Cow-pox Mange', the phenomenon of the 'Ox-faced Boy' and the like – there was in their diatribes hardly a mention of syphilis. John Birch, another of Jenner's critics, quoting the observation of a pro-vaccinationist that 'the vaccine disease is some pollution imposed upon the harmless animal by the milker', asked 'what that disease is which [...] produces the vaccine matter? Is it the Itch? the Lues Venera [i.e. venereal disease] or the Small-Pox itself?' Birch, however, takes the matter no further. Joseph Adams, Physician to the Small-Pox and Inoculation Hospitals, in a pamphlet giving practical advice on carrying out vaccination (1807), stressed that the subject from whom 'virus' was taken should be healthy, 'though it is not likely that any other disease should be inoculated with the variolous', and this seems to have been the accepted medical opinion for the next fifty years or so. Gregory (1838) suggested that the fears of parents did not, for the most part, go beyond scrofula, the King's evil.

A striking shift of emphasis occurred with the introduction in 1853 of compulsion, which focused attention sharply on the source of the 'vaccine disease'. Even private vaccinators had to vaccinate with cowpox, but the parents could choose the source from which the lymph was derived. Parents dependent on the state service could exercise no control over the selection of the vaccinifer, which was made by the public vaccinator from the arms available at his station and could include those of the offspring of some of the poorest, least healthy and least hygienic families in the neighbourhood. John Gibbs, in his impassioned letter to the President of the Board of Health, asked why vaccination was held in horror by so many parents. It was because of the thought that a disease, loathsome in itself, was to be transmitted to their children 'through they know not how many unhealthy mediums: they have a dread, a conviction, that other filthy diseases, tending to embitter and shorten life, are frequently transmitted through and by a vaccine virus'.

In his *Vaccination Papers*, issued in the following year, John Simon emphatically rejected the anti-vaccinationists' allegations: 'I must say that I believe it to be utterly impossible, except under gross and punishable misconduct, for any other infection than that of cowpox to be communicated in what pretends to be the performance of vaccination.' In support of his contention he set out in tabular form the replies he had received from '542 members of my own profession, at home and abroad' to the question:

Have you any reason to believe that lymph, from a true Jennerian vesicle, has ever been a vehicle of syphilitic, scrophulous or other constitutional infection to the vaccinated person; or that unintentional inoculation with some other disease, instead of the proper vaccination, has occurred in the hands of a duly educated medical practitioner?[4]

The answers, as regarded syphilitic inoculation, were 'only just short of being an absolutely uniform NO'.

At least one other leading authority delivered a verdict equally uncompromising. In his *Handbook of Vaccination* (1868) Seaton (probably Simon's closest associate) dealt at some length with the 'allegation' that syphilis might be 'invaccinated'. This was not supported, he claimed, by general professional experience, nor by pathological considerations, nor by experiment: 'Of course, insertion of the matter of syphilis will produce syphilis. The harmlessness of vaccination is dependent on due care being used.'[5] Suppose there existed risks of vaccino-syphilitic inoculation: what, after all, did those risks amount to? 'During the eight years in which there has been systematic inspection of public vaccination in England some millions of vaccinations have been performed: but the inspectors have no knowledge of any such accident having occurred in any one instance.' Within three years that claim could no longer be made.

Unlike smallpox, syphilis had a fairly clearly defined history as a European disease. It was generally held to have been imported from the West Indies at the end of the fifteenth century by the returning ships of Christopher Columbus, after which, in the words of one of its historians, 'it ran a virulent course until about 1600, when it settled down into an endemic risk attendant upon dissolute living'. By the mid-nineteenth century it was in no sense a scourge on the same scale as smallpox. In 1858, according to Farr, it killed 1,006 persons in England and Wales, 'in a large portion infants, who had received it as their only inheritance'.[6] A few years later he recorded 'a marked increase of deaths referred to syphilis', and in 1875 that it was 'twice as fatal in the five years 1870–1874 as it was twenty years ago. Of nearly 2,000 deaths ascribed to syphilis [in 1874] 1,484 were babies under one year of age'.

It was in 1871, when the great smallpox pandemic was at its height and the select committee was conducting its inquiry into the Vaccination Acts, that facts were made known that, in the words of the expert who revealed them, 'produced in the British [medical] profession a sense of most disagreeable surprise and awoke many for the first time to the perception of a danger which they had never before realized and which most had scarcely credited'. No one can have been more disagreeably surprised than John Simon.

In March of that year there occurred what, in a somewhat casual understatement, he described as 'a curious chapter of accidents'. One week after he had given evidence to the select committee, the Medical Department of the Privy Council, which Seaton was temporarily presiding over, learned of some suspected 'cases of co-infection of syphilitic cow-pox'. Seaton immediately sought advice from an independent expert described in his obituary in 1913 as 'for many years the first English authority on syphilis'. At the time of the incident Jonathan Hutchinson was senior surgeon to the London Hospital, surgeon to the Moorfields Ophthalmic Hospital and to the Hospital for Skin Diseases. In due course he became President of the Royal College of Surgeons. A firm believer in compulsory vaccination, he was one of the respondents to Simon's questionnaire who had contributed to the 'almost absolutely uniform NO'.

The initial stages of the case, as described by Hutchinson, offer an interesting glimpse of the relationship, at a practical level, between public vaccinators and private practitioners:

> On February 7th 1871 a young surgeon [i.e. not a public vacci-nator] applied to a public vaccine station for a supply of lymph. He was offered a healthy looking infant of four months old, then in the eighth day [since her own vaccination] and with five good vesicles. As he wished to vaccinate a considerable number of persons in the same house he preferred to borrow the child rather than, as at first proposed, to charge points [with lymph], and arrangements having been made with the mother [i.e. in return for an agreed fee] the child was at once taken to a private house where eleven young adults (shopmen and servants) were vacci-nated from its arm.[7]

Only four (of the five) vesicles were used, and more than one of them 'bled somewhat'. Two further vaccinations were afterwards performed with lymph from the same source: thirteen vaccinations from one child. All but one of them, which did not 'take', passed off without incident and were at first regarded as successful, until about two months later, when, after the scars had again become sore, it was 'quite certain that ten of the twelve vaccinees had indurated chancres on their arms' – the first and certain signs of acquired syphilis.

The vaccinifer had gone through her own vaccination without incident and appeared healthy, but on examining her Hutchinson discovered the symptoms of syphilis. There was not the slightest reason, he wrote, for thinking that the disease had been introduced into the child's system at the time of her own vaccination: the symptoms and the course of the disease would have been entirely different. This was constitutional syphilis, inherited from the mother, and there was little doubt in Hutchinson's mind that 'it was the blood and not the vaccine lymph, which was the source of the disease' in the ten cases he was investigating. There was no reason to suppose that any of the patients had suffered from syphilis in the past, and they all subsequently recovered after the usual treatment.

While Hutchinson was still investigating these occurrences he was asked by a colleague to inspect two children on whom syphilitic eruptions had appeared seven weeks after their vaccination. Further inquiry showed that out of 24 other children vaccinated from the same vaccinifer, at the same session, nine had the tell-tale chancres on their arms and a further six were 'suffering from well-marked and copious rashes'. The vaccinifer was now seven months old, and apparently well grown and healthy, but on examination showed unmistakable signs of syphilis.

The chief conclusion to be drawn from these events was that the precaution stressed by all writers on the subject as paramount – the avoidance of taking blood when opening a vesicle to obtain lymph – was being either ignored or at best breached inadvertently by insufficiently skilful operators. (A witness later told the Royal Commission on Vaccination that in his opinion it was impossible to avoid taking blood.)

To the anti-vaccinationists all discussion of causes was irrelevant: it was the consequence that mattered. *Vaccination Tract No. 7* asked: 'If seven infants die every week of syphilis in London how many are there left alive with the same disease? How many of these are ignorantly vaccinated from? What is the natural increase of syphilis thus [...] and how long will it take to extend the poison of syphilis to the entire population?' A certain Dr Richardson asserted in *Good Words* (1876) that syphilis 'leaves its imprint more or less on every hundredth babe at least born in this kingdom and engrafts a host of maladies on half our Saxon race'. Taking this statement as a basis, George S. Gibbs, a relation of John and Fellow of the Statistical Society, constructed tables showing that

> It is a moderate estimate that for every diseased child used as a source of lymph ten others will be diseased, and if we allow the vaccinators sufficient acumen to reject one half of these unfortu- nates [...] we shall then have the disease spread among the children of London [...] at an average rate of 4,000 per annum and in the whole of England at the rate of 35,000 per annum...[8]

Vaccination Tract No. 8, given over entirely to 'The Propagation of Syphilis to Infants and Adults by Vaccination and Re-vaccination', quoted from a report in the *Medical Times and Gazette* (February 1873):

> As the law stands infants must be vaccinated before they are three months old: but, apart from snuffles [an early indication of syphilis] there may be no manifestation of constitutional syphilis till they are six or eight months old, or even it may be later [...] It is quite plain from past experience that heifer vaccination cannot be kept up, save in times of public excitement, except the Govern- ment intervene, and it is not fair to subject people's children to risks such as those which vaccination-syphilis implies, with no alternative save to go to prison.

The medical and political establishments had little difficulty in brushing aside the apocalyptic forecasts of their wilder opponents, but appear to have recognized that the arm-to-arm method of vaccination, so long the foundation of the entire system, had been undermined by Hutchinson's cases and that if the whole edifice were not eventually to collapse under the onslaught of public opinion some alternative must be found to the use of 'humanized' lymph, as it was frequently described; in other words, the human vaccinifer must ultimately be eliminated from the process.

The obvious alternative had been under investigation on the conti- nent for some years under the slightly misleading description 'animal vaccination', implying the use of lymph taken directly from the calf that had been inoculated with cowpox. There were drawbacks to the operation, but medical men on the continent had continued their experiments, and only two years before Hutchinson delivered his verdicts Seaton had been despatched to various locations in Europe – Paris, Brussels and Rotterdam among others – to observe and report on the latest developments. He returned convinced that there was no foreseeable future for animal vaccination, which had disadvantages 'of such a kind as at present to forbid [its] adoption in place of our own'.[9] This view prevailed for nearly a decade: according to the Annual Report of the Local Government Board for 1869 an investigation into 'the effects upon children of lymph derived from the Animal Vaccination Institution of Brussels' showed that there was no reason for preferring the results of calf lymph. The National Vaccine Establishment, happily sending out its thousands of charges of dried humanized vaccine every year, showed little interest in new continental developments.

Nevertheless, as the *Lancet* pointed out in July 1879, important changes had been taking place among sections of the medical profession and the public that the Local Government Board had not been 'quite alive to'. The drawbacks that Seaton had pointed out were said to have been entirely removed, and animal vaccination could be performed 'with as much certainty as with humanized lymph'.

In an attempt, presumably, to induce a greater sense of urgency, four prominent Members of Parliament, including Lyon Playfair, promoted in 1879 and again in 1880 a 'Bill to Encourage Vaccination by providing facilities for the optional use of Animal Vaccination'. It proposed that if parents required to have a child vaccinated should stipulate the use of animal lymph 'it shall be the duty of the public vaccinators so to vaccinate, and to do so in all cases where it was their duty to vaccinate gratuitously'. The Local Government Board would be required to take measures, at the public expense, to 'secure for the public a supply of animal lymph and to provide for its distribution to public vaccinators and medical practitioners within the United Kingdom'.

The Bill was not proceeded with but appears to have had the desired effect. The Registrar General's report covering the year 1879 noted that 'we have had under consideration the question whether it might be desirable [...] to make arrangements for a supply of lymph from the calf as well as from the human subject'. There would be obvious difficulties in carrying out a scheme using calf lymph for every one of the 700,000 to 800,000 vaccinations performed every year; the proposal therefore was 'to supplement with calf lymph the resources of the [National Vaccine] Establishment'. Within two or three years premises for the new service had been found in London, calf-to-calf vaccination was being carried out and a steadily increasing supply of lymph was being produced. By 1882 the Establishment was sending out dried calf lymph 'for the commencement of a local service of arm-to-arm vaccinations with instructions on how to overcome some of the disadvantages as compared with humanized lymph'. Any doubts were dispelled by the Annual Report for 1885 of the Medical Officer of the Local Government Board: 'The success of calf-vaccination on children has been all that could be desired [...] and has been practically identical with that of vaccination with humanized lymph in the hands of the same operators.'

One further step was needed. It had been known for some years that the amount of lymph available for vaccination could be considerably increased if a given quantity were diluted by three times its bulk of glycerine, and that the mixture appeared to keep as well as did unmixed lymph. A method of overcoming a drawback to the process was proposed by two British scientists, Drs Copeman and Bloxall. The Royal Commission's final report looked favourably on the discovery, subject to further investigation, and this, taken in conjunction with the observation in the preceding paragraph of the report – 'We think that vaccine vesicles should not be opened unless for some adequate reason' – seemed to spell the end of the arm-to-arm transmission of humanized lymph almost exactly a century after Jenner had inaugurated it.

PART III

The Retreat from Compulsion

CHAPTER 19

A GENUINE CONSCIENTIOUS OBJECTION

Although no legislation on the subject of vaccination was enacted between 1871 and 1898, apart from the short Act of 1874, which was designed to clarify the Act of 1871, the anti-vaccination movement continued to bring the opposition to compulsion before the House of Commons, concentrating mainly at first on the question of repeated penalties for default. Three attempts in six years to amend the law 'so far as accumulating penalties are concerned' made no progress. There was considerable astonishment and derision when in 1880 J. G. Dodson, President of the Local Government Board in Gladstone's second administration, appeared to be doing the anti-vaccinationists' work for them by introducing a Bill to limit penalties, virtually along the lines of its predecessors. The *Lancet* explained that although it was generally regarded as 'a Bill for the evasion of vaccination' it had in reality 'a different and more commendable object – namely the abatement of the nuisance of the so-called "vaccination martyrs"'. The *Lancet* was prepared to support the Bill: 'Take away the element of "martyrdom" and interest in these self-cultivated sufferers will collapse [...] Conscientious parents will continue to put their faith in vaccination.' This degree of confidence was not widely shared and when the medical profession threatened all-out opposition to a 'bill for promoting smallpox' Dodson withdrew it.

The leading anti-vaccinationists now decided to change their tactics and demand total repeal of the compulsory clauses of the Acts, not in the hope of achieving it at this stage but with the intention of arousing public interest and inducing the government to set up a Royal Commission to investigate the whole subject. In 1883 a Bill to repeal the compulsory clauses gave rise to a debate that roused the Commons from its customary torpor where vaccination was concerned.[1] Thanks largely to a vigorous speech from the government side by Lyon Playfair the motion was rejected by 264 votes to 18. Yet only two years later the great Leicester demonstration showed the extent of public support that the movement could call on. Its growing strength became more obvious still in the late 1880s when a smallpox epidemic in Sheffield, generally regarded as 'a well-vaccinated city', resulted in 600 deaths in a matter of months.[2] A very thorough investigation produced no satisfactory explanation of the severity of the outbreak, except for a telling observation of the Lord Mayor that in spite of past efforts the city had no system, such as existed in Leicester, which required medical men to inform the authorities immediately of any case of smallpox that occurred so that the victim could be promptly and totally isolated to prevent the spread of infection. The anti-vaccinationists capitalized on the outbreak in Sheffield by demanding that the Home Secretary appoint a Royal Commission, and in what has been described as a volte-face (possibly influenced by events in Sheffield) the President of the Local Government Board, Henry Chaplin, granted the request, not, he insisted, 'because [the government] have the slightest doubt of the efficiency of vaccination, but because the state of public opinion requires that a thorough investigation should be made into the whole question'.

The Commission, which began its sittings in 1889, was instructed to inquire and report on:

1) The effect of vaccination in reducing the prevalence of, and the mortality from, smallpox.

2) What means, other than vaccination, can be used for diminishing the prevalence of smallpox, and how far such means could be relied on in the place of vaccination.

3) The objections made to vaccination on the ground of injurious effects alleged to result therefrom; and the nature and extent of any injurious effects which do, in fact, so result.

4) Whether any, and, if so, what means should be adopted for preventing or lessening the ill effects, if any, resulting from vaccination; and whether, and, if so, by what means, vaccination with animal vaccine should be further facilitated as part of public vaccination.

5) Whether any alterations should be made in the arrangements for securing the performance of vaccination, and, in particular, in the provisions of the Vaccination Acts with respect to prosecutions for non-compliance with the law.[3]

The investigation of these issues was thorough beyond anything that was likely to have been foreseen. Chaired by Lord Herschell, a former Lord Chief Justice, at the head of a formidable array of medical and legal authorities, and with prominent anti-vaccinationists led by W. J. Collins, the Commission took seven years to complete its task (sitting, it is true, only on Wednesday afternoons, with long vacations). Nearly 200 witnesses gave evidence, on both sides of the argument, often at inordinate length, as when during almost three sessions no member of the Commission uttered a word while a leading opponent of vaccination from Leicester took them step by step through 51 tables of statistics, allegedly proving the ineffectiveness of vaccination.

The most notable event during the seemingly interminable inquiry occurred with the publication of the fifth of the Commission's annual interim reports, which broke away from the laconic one-sentence format of its predecessors 'to make recommendations with respect to certain subsidiary questions to which our attention has been drawn'.[4] The first recommendation, which could be said to arise from the fifth of the questions set out in the Commission's remit, recalled the events of 1871 by virtually accepting the conclusion of the select committee of that year embodied in the clause that the House of Lords had succeeded in removing from the ensuing Act. The Royal Commission's recommendation was that 'the imposition of repeated penalties in respect of the non-vaccination of the same child should no longer be possible'. The justification given for the change was that 'any advantage which may arise from the tendency of repeated convictions to increase vaccination is more than counterbalanced by the resentment and active opposition to vaccination which they engender'.

The second recommendation addressed a more serious abuse – the treatment of parents who, having refused or been unable to pay fines, had been given a prison sentence. Accounts of their experiences, even allowing for some excusable exaggeration, revealed regimes of severity and harshness that were out of all proportion to the offence, and were due, in the Commission's opinion, to a deliberate misreading by the Home Secretary of the Prisons Act, which stated explicitly that '[i]n a prison where debtors are confined means shall be provided for separating them altogether from the criminal prisoners'. The Home Secretary had decided that this should not apply to those imprisoned under the Vaccination Acts for non-payment of fines. The Commission now recommended firmly that 'persons imprisoned under the Vaccination Acts should no longer be subjected to the same treatment as criminals', but should be treated as 'simple imprisonment prisoners', and were therefore 'not to be sentenced to hard labour'. The Commissioners' reasoning was that 'many of those whose imprisonment arises from the contravention of the laws relating to vaccination regard the practice as likely to be injurious to the health of their children, and are well conducted and in other respects law-abiding citizens'. Subjecting them to the treatment awarded to criminals was not 'calculated to secure obedience to the law or to add to the number of the vaccinated'.

Both recommendations, although rationally defended and based on more than thirty years' experience of the failure of the existing system, were predictably and bitterly attacked by hardliners in the compulsion camp, but for those shrewd enough to read between the lines they provided a clear pointer to the spirit of the conclusions that the Commission was likely to reach in its final report. Owing to confusion among the anti-vaccinationist leaders, and an unfortunately timed change of government, a Bill that was intended to give effect to the Commission's recommendations made no progress.

The Commission's final report was issued in 1896 (with a dissenting report written by Collins and J. A. Picton, a Methodist minister who, as the anti-vaccinationist candidate at a by-election in 1884, had been returned unopposed as one of Leicester's two MPs). It offered something less than the anti-vaccination lobby had hoped for and far more than the pro-compulsion medical and political establishments had expected to have to concede. It made numerous recommendations, of which the main ones were that vaccination should continue to be compulsory but that parents who could demonstrate a conscientious objection to having the operation carried out on a child should not be compelled to do so. This concession, as was furiously pointed out, could and probably would undermine the whole purpose of the Vaccination Acts. How, for example, could magistrates who would have to decide the issue tell whether the parent had a genuine conscientious objection?

A Bill incorporating most of the Commission's proposal but not the significant concession of a conscience clause was introduced by Henry Chaplin. After a great deal of political infighting and bargaining a compromise proposed by Balfour, which stopped short only of the abolition of compulsion, secured the passage of the Vaccination Act of 1898. By a remarkable irony this argument took place against the background of the last major epidemic of smallpox to occur in Britain. Under the leadership of the proprietor of a local newspaper the city of Gloucester had almost completely abandoned vaccination, until 1896, when an outbreak of smallpox in one area spread rapidly, as much as anything because facilities for dealing with it were grossly inadequate.[5] Unabashed, the leading opponents of vaccination continued their campaign (which was based largely on the familiar contention that smallpox was not infectious but a 'filth' disease) but towards the end of March 1896 the Gloucester Union decided to enforce the requirements of the existing Vaccination Acts and the number of vaccinations in the city rose swiftly.

The nationwide battle against compulsion was by no means over, largely because of the unwillingness of magistrates to accept protestations from 'conscientious objectors', but after much activity by the National Anti-Vaccination League, coupled with the electoral swing that produced the Liberal government of 1906, an Act was passed in 1907 that, by allowing a dissenting parent to make a 'statutory declaration' instead of having to persuade a magistrate to issue a certificate of exemption, effectively brought compulsion to an end. Smallpox itself declined sharply as an epidemic disease until it became virtually unknown in Britain, but the Acts that in theory continued to make vaccination compulsory remained on the statute book until as late as 1946, when the National Health and Insurance Act stipulated that 'The Vaccination Acts [...] shall [...] cease to have effect'.

If there is a lesson to be learnt from this well-documented but almost totally unremarked history of legislation, which in its time affected the life of every family, and indeed of every child born in Britain, it is perhaps to be found in a comment made by the Royal Commission:

Too blind a confidence is sometimes reposed in the power of an Act of Parliament [...] When that which the law enjoins imposes on parents the duty of a performance which they [...] regard as prejudicial to their children the very attempt to compel obedience may defeat the object of the legislation.[6]

This remark, invoked by specific legislation, might not have been needed if a similar warning in more general terms, given by William Farr, had been heeded. In 1843, ten years before the Act inaugurating compulsory vaccination was passed, Farr, a passionate advocate of the operation, wrote: 'care must be taken to discriminate between what can be done by legislation for the people, and what can only be accomplished by themselves individually and swayed by the slow progress of opinion'.[7]

NOTES

1 The Byzantine Operation

1 Wharncliffe (ed.), *Letters and Works of Lady Mary Wortley Montagu with Introductory Anecdotes by Lady Louisa Stuart*, 1837, p. 308.
2 R. Halsband, 'New light on Lady Mary Wortley Montagu's contribution to inoculation', *Journal of the History of Medicine*, VIII, 1953, p. 394.
3 Quoted in C. W. Dixon, *Smallpox*, 1962, p. 221.

2 The Small Pockes

1 C. Creighton, *The History of Epidemics in Britain*, 2 vols, 1965 (repr.), vol. 1, p. 446.
2 H. A. L. Fisher, *A History of Europe*, 1936, p. 137.
3 Lucretius, *De Rerum Natura/On the Nature of the Universe* (trans. Latham), 1951, p. 28.
4 Lucretius, *De Rerum Natura*, p. 250.
5 Sydenham, *Life and Original Writings*, p. 104.
6 W. Wagstaffe, *A letter to Dr Freind shewing the danger and uncertainty of inoculating the small pox*, 1722, p. 7.
7 J. Moore, *A reply to the Anti-vaccinists*, 1806, p. 37.
8 Moore, *A reply*, p. 8.
9 D. Baxby, *Jenner's Smallpox Vaccine: the Riddle of Vaccinia Virus and its Origin*, 1981, p. 20.
10 G. Miller, *The Adoption of Inoculation*, 1957, p. 26.
11 W. Watson, *An Account of a Series of Experiments with a View to ascertaining the most successful Method of inoculating the Small Pox*, 1768, p. 38
12 C. Tomalin, *Jane Austen, A Life*, 1997, p. 126.
13 W. Holland, *Paupers and Pig Killers*, 1994, p. 8.
14 Dixon, *Smallpox*, p. 107.

3 The Engrafted Distemper

1 For a full account see Dixon, *Smallpox*, p. 338.
2 I. Grundy, *Lady Mary Wortley Montagu*, 1999, p. 211; G. Miller, 'Putting Lady Mary

Wortley Montagu in her Place', *Bulletin of Medical History*, 1981, p. 78.
3 H. Sloane, *An Account of Inoculation* (Philosophical Transactions, xlix), 1756, p. 516.
4 Wharncliffe (ed.), *Letters and Works*, p. 89.
5 Halsband, 'New light'.

4 The Language of Figures

1 J. Jurin, *An Account of the Success of Inoculating the Small Pox in Great Britain with a Comparison between the Miscarriage in the Practice and the Mortality of the Natural Small Pox*, 1724.
2 W. White, *The Story of a Great Delusion*, 1885, p. 78.
3 G. Jenner, *The evidence at large as laid before the Committee of the House of Commons respecting Dr Jenner's discovery of Vaccine Inoculation, and the debate which followed*, 1805, p. 33.
4 Jenner, *The evidence at large*, p. 86.
5 R. M. MacLeod, *Law, Medicine and Public Opinion: The Resistance to Compulsory Health Legislation 1870–1907*, Public Law 1967, p. 111; Dixon, *Smallpox*, p. 288.

5 The Suttonian System

1 T. Fosbrooke, 'Biographical Anecdotes of Dr Jenner', *Berkeley Manuscripts*, 1821, p. 221.
2 I. Maddox, *A Sermon Preached at St. Andrews, Holborn*, 1752; W. Woodville, *The History of the Inoculation of the Small-pox in Great Britain*, 1796, p. 238.
3 The Declaration was, of course, written in Latin, and has been translated more than once in various styles. I have remained with Woodville's version as conveying the authentic eighteenth-century flavour.
4 G. M. Trevelyan, *English Social History*, 1942, p. 293.
5 J. Moore, *History of Smallpox and Inoculation*, 1815, p. 303.
6 T. Dimsdale, *Thoughts on General and Partial Inoculation*, 1776, p. 10.
7 Dimsdale, *Thoughts*, p. 205.
8 Dimsdale, *Thoughts*, p. 55.
9 T. Dimsdale, *The Present Method of Inoculating for the Smallpox*, 1767, p. 39.
10 Dimsdale, *Present Method*, p. 83.
11 D. Sutton, *The Inoculator, or Suttonian System of Inoculation*, 1796, p. 60.
12 T. Dimsdale, *Observations on the Introduction to the Plan of a Dispensary for a General Inoculation*, 1788, p. 54.
13 Dimsdale, *Thoughts*, p. 24.
14 Dimsdale, *Thoughts*, p. 123.
15 J. Haygarth, *An Inquiry how to prevent the Small Pox*, 1777, p. 85.
16 Haygarth, *An Inquiry*, p. 118.
17 Haygarth, *An Inquiry*, p. 481.
18 But see Hough (1737) 'parents are tender and fearful, not without hope that their children may escape this disease, or have it favourably, whereas in the way of art, should it prove fatal they would never forgive themselves.' Quoted in Dixon, *Smallpox*, p. 348.
19 J. Haygarth, *A Sketch of a Plan to Exterminate the Casual Smallpox*, 1793, p. 128.

20 Haygarth, *A Sketch of a Plan*, p. vii.
21 Haygarth, *A Sketch of a Plan*, p. 116.
22 Jenner, *The evidence at large*, p. 32.
23 Quoted in Simon, *Vaccination Papers*, p. x.
24 Quoted in White, *Story of a Great Delusion*, p. 53.
25 Creighton, *History of Epidemics*, vol. 2, p. 512.

6 The Great Benefactor

1 J. Baron, *The Life of Edward Jenner* (2 vols), 1838, p. 123.
2 Baron, *Life of Edward Jenner*, p. 138.
3 Baron, *Life of Edward Jenner*, p. 580.
4 Baron, *Life of Edward Jenner*, p. 7.
5 See Fosbrooke, 'Biographical Anecdotes', quoted in Fisher, *History of Europe*, p. 29.
6 This early promise was unfortunately deceptive; the boy was never strong and died of consumption in 1810.
7 Baron, *Life of Edward Jenner*, p. 128.
8 Baron, *Life of Edward Jenner*, p. 134.
9 E. Seaton, *A Handbook of Vaccination*, 1868, p. 198.
10 Baron, *Life of Edward Jenner*, p. 367.
11 Baron, *Life of Edward Jenner*, p. 490.
12 An advertisement published in the *Morning Herald*, quoted in B. Moseley, *A Treatise on the Lues Bovilla, or Cow-pox*, 1805, p. 14.
13 Cobbett, 'Advice to a Father on Vaccination', quoted in *Vaccination Tract No. 3*, p. 6.
14 Baron, *Life of Edward Jenner*, vol. 2, p. 362.
15 Pearson to Jenner, quoted in Baron, *Life of Edward Jenner*, p. 305.
16 Baron, *Life of Edward Jenner*, p. 319.
17 Baron, *Life of Edward Jenner*, p. 320.
18 Baxby, *Jenner's Smallpox Vaccine*.
19 Baron, *Life of Edward Jenner*, p. 491.
20 J. Ring, *A Caution against Vaccination Swindlers and Imposters*, p. 35.
21 Baron, *Life of Edward Jenner*, p. 192.
22 Baron, *Life of Edward Jenner*, vol. 2, p. 303.
23 Baron, *Life of Edward Jenner*, vol. 2, p. 311.

7 The Speckled Monster

1 Quoted in Simon, *Vaccination Papers*, App. C, p. 4.
2 Simon, *Vaccination Papers*, p. 6.
3 Baron, *Life of Edward Jenner*, vol. 2, p. 56.
4 Simon, *Vaccination Papers*, App. p. 8.
5 Letter from Jenner to Lettsom, quoted in J. Ring, *Treatise on the cow-pox*, 1801–03, p. 864.
6 Baron, *Life of Edward Jenner*, p. 72.
7 *Edinburgh Review*, January 1810.
8 *Lancet*, 9 March 1867, p. 304.
9 Ring, *Treatise*, p. 8.

10 I. Lettsom, *Observations On the Cow-Pock*, 1801, quoted in Ring, *Treatise*, p. 859.
11 Ring, *Treatise*, p. 2.
12 Moore, *A Reply*, p. 8.
13 Baron, *Life of Edward Jenner*, p. 269.
14 J. Crosse, *A History of the Variolous Epidemic which occurred in Norwich in the Year 1819*, 1820, p. 11.

8 The Three Bashaws

1 S. and B. Webb, *English Local Government: English Poor History: The Last Hundred Years*, vol. 1, 1929, p. 81: 'a bureaucratic authority, acting by its own volition, without request from, or consent of, any local inhabitants, without even ratification by the House of Commons, without any chance of appeal.'
2 Transactions of PMSA 25/7/1838: report of section appointed to inquire into the state of vaccination, p. 90.
3 Official circulars of the Poor Law Commissioners, vol. 7, no. 5, 1 May 1847.
4 T. Malthus, *An Essay on the Principle of Population*, 1798, rev. edn 1830.
5 H. W. Rumsey, *Essays on State Medicine*, 1856, p. 182.
6 PLC official circular, 1 September 1840.
7 1st Report to Registrar General, letter from William Farr, App. P.
8 W. Farr, 'Note on the Present Epidemic of Smallpox', *The Lancet*, 28 November 1840, p. 353.

9 A Competent and Energetic Officer

1 Quoted in Rumsey, *Essays on State Medicine*, p. 133.
2 See Bibliography, Parliamentary Papers.
3 *Report*, p. 21.
4 *Memorial presented to the President of the Board of Health*, Parliamentary Papers.
5 *Memorial*.
6 J. Simon, *English Sanitary Institutions*, 1890, p. 259.
7 This appears to be inaccurate. The same Bill was introduced twice in 1856. No Bill was introduced in 1857.
8 President of the General Board of Health (later Lord Mount Temple).
9 J. R. Hutchinson, *A Historical Note on the Prevention of Smallpox*, 1946–47.
10 R. Lambert, *Sir John Simon*, 1963, p. 256.
11 Simon, *English Sanitary Institutions*, p. 261.
12 Marson, *Petition*, quoted in Simon, *Vaccination Papers*, App. G., p. 26.
13 Simon, *Vaccination Papers*, p. lxx.
14 Simon, *Vaccination Papers*, p. lxxvi.

10 Formidable Men

1 N. Annan, *Leslie Stephen: The Godless Victorian*, 1984, p. 13.
2 Simon, *English Sanitary Institutions*, p. 232.
3 Lambert, *Sir John Simon*, p. 257.

4 Lambert, *Sir John Simon*, p. 357.
5 Simon, *English Sanitary Institutions*, p. 281.
6 Simon, *English Sanitary Institutions*, p. 285.

11 The Present Non-System

1 6th Report of the Medical Officer to the Privy Council, p. 156.
2 6th Report, p. 88.
3 4th Report, p. 59.
4 *Lancet*, 9 April 1853, p. 344.
5 Marson quoted in Simon, 'Vaccination Papers', App. F, p. 22.
6 6th Report, p. 140.
7 6th Report, p. 142.
8 4th Report, p. 72.
9 6th Report, p. 219.
10 5th Report, p. 109.
11 4th Report, p. 63.
12 Report of MO to the Privy Council and the Local Government Board for 1875 [c 1318], p. 92.
13 S. M. Copeman, 'Vaccination', *Encyclopedia Britannica*, 11th edn, 1911, p. 833.
14 *Lancet*, 8 June 1867, p. 721.
15 6th Report of the Registrar General 1844, p. xiii.
16 'The Journeyman Engineer' (Thomas Wright), *The Great Unwashed*, 1868 (repr. 1970) p. 259.
17 6th Report, p. 145.

12 *Toties Quoties*

1 *Pilcher v. Stafford*: for a full account see D. P. Fry, *The Law Relating to Vaccination*, 1872, p. 93.
2 Hansard (Commons), 14 June 1867, col. 1868.
3 Seaton, *Handbook*, p. 396.
4 *Allen v. Worthy*: See Fry, *Law Relating to Vaccination*, p. 163.

13 Crotchety People

1 Report of Select Committee, 1871, p. 13.
2 U. Bright, *An evil law unfairly enforced*, 1886.
3 Report of Select Committee, Q.1343.
4 Report, Q.2521.
5 Report, Q.4174.
6 Report, Q.4509.
7 Report, Q.3315.
8 Report, Q.3318.
9 Report, Q.3319.
10 Report, Q.3323.

11 Report, Q.3338.
12 Report, Q.3330.
13 Report, Q.3439.
14 Report, Q.3443.
15 Report, Q.61.
16 Simon, *English Sanitary Institutions*, p. 311.
17 *BMJ*, 7 February 1874, p. 178.
18 Simon, *English Sanitary Institutions*, p. 347(f/n).
19 Hansard, Vol. 208, Vacc. Amendment Bill (191), col. 1708, 15 August 1871.
20 Hansard, 18 August 1871, col. 1843.
21 Hansard (Commons), 19 August 1871.

14 A Loathsome Virus

1 J. Gibbs, Esq., letter to the President of the Board of Health, entitled 'Compulsory Vaccination, briefly considered in its scientific, religious and political aspects'; 1856 (109) LII.489.
2 H. Pitman, *Prison Thoughts on Vaccination*, 1877.
3 Letter dated 7 July 1869, reprinted from *The Co-operator*.
4 *Vaccination Tract No.5*, p. 4.
5 E. S. Tokswig, *Swedenborg, Scientist and Mystic*, 1949, p. 96.
6 Quoted in White, *Story of a Great Delusion*, p. 549.
7 *Vaccination Tract No.7*, p. 9.

15 A Cruel and Degrading Imposture

1 P. Razzell, 'Edward Jenner: the History of a Medical Myth', *Medical History*, 1965, 9, pp. 216–29. See also Baxby, *Jenner's Smallpox Vaccine*, pp. 104–11.
2 E. M. Crookshank, *The History and Pathology of Vaccination* (2 vols), 1889, vol. 1, p. 463.
3 Crookshank, *History and Pathology*, vol. 1, p. 464.
4 C. Creighton, *Jenner and Vaccination*, 1889, p. 48.
5 A. Hirsch, *Handbook of geographical and historical pathology*, 1883, p. 141.
6 W. White, *Swedenborg, His Life and Times*, 1867, p. 664.
7 T. Frewen, *The Practice and Theory of Inoculation*, 1749, p. 14.
8 W. Langton, *An Address to the Public on the present Method of Inoculation*, 1767, p. 12.
9 Woodville, *History*, p. 33.
10 G. Blane, *A statement of facts tending to establish an estimate of the true value and present state of vaccination*, 1820, p. 14.
11 Simon, *Vaccination Papers*, p. ix.
12 Royal Commission Report, p. 96.
13 G. Wilson, *The Hazards of Immunisation*, 1962, p. 7.
14 Jenner quoted by White, *Story of a Great Delusion*, p. 112.
15 White, *Story of a Great Delusion*, p. 112.
16 White, *Story of a Great Delusion*, p. 119; but see Baxby, *Jenner's Smallpox Vaccine*, p. 75: 'I think it is fair to conclude that the evidence in the "Inquiry" although not extensive, was sound and probably sufficient to justify his main claim.'

17 White, *Story of a Great Delusion*, p. 124.
18 White, *Story of a Great Delusion*, p. xlviii.
19 Dixon, *Smallpox*, p. 256.
20 D. Baxby, 'Edward Jenner, William Woodville and the Origins of Vaccinia Virus', *Journal of the History of Medicine*, April 1979, p. 162.
21 M. Holroyd, *Bernard Shaw: The Search for Love, 1856–1898*, 1988, p. 92.
22 G. B. Shaw,' Preface', *The Doctor's Dilemma*, 1906, p. 27.
23 T. Dimsdale, *Tracts on Inoculation*, 1781, p. 144.
24 Haygarth, *A Sketch of a Plan*, p. 59.
25 White, *Story of a Great Delusion*, p. 174.

16 Ten Shillings or Seven Days

1 J. D. Rolleston, 'The Smallpox Pandemic of 1870–74', *Proceedings of the Royal Society of Medicine 1933–34*, 27, 1; E. Seaton, 'Report on the Recent Epidemic of Smallpox in the United Kingdom in relation to Vaccination and the Vaccination Laws', *Annual Report to the Local Government Board [c.1318]*, 1875.
2 *Lancet*, 17 June 1871, p. 833.
3 Report of Select Committee, 1871, p. 14.
4 Vaccination Prosecutions, copy of letter from the Local Government Board to guardians of Evesham Union etc.
5 Papers relative to the prosecution of defaulters.
6 MacLeod, *Law, Medicine and Public Opinion*, p. 125.
7 *Leicester Mercury*, 6 May 1884.
8 *Leicester Mercury*, 10 August 1884.
9 *Leicester Mercury*, 3 August 1884.
10 *Leicester Mercury*, 10 June 1884.
11 *Leicester Mercury*, 30 January 1884.
12 *Leicester Mercury*, 24 March 1885.

17 Death by Non-Vaccination

1 4th Report of the Local Government Board 1884/85, Supplement [C4516].
2 Report of the Select Committee on the Office of Coroner, 30 March 1860 (193).
3 4th Annual Report of the Registrar General, Appendix [423], 1842. Nosology is the branch of medicine which deals with the classification of diseases.
4 *Lancet*, 9 March 1867, p. 303.
5 Report of the Select Committee, Q.1963.
6 Instructions for Vaccinators under Contract: 16th Annual Report of the Local Government Board, 1886–87 [c.5171], p. 39.
7 Mr Radcliffe's report was published.
8 Report to the President of the Local Government Board into certain deaths and injuries... at Norwich, 1882.
9 W. J. Collins, *A Review of the Norwich Vaccination Inquiry*, read at the monthly conference of the London Society for the Abolition of Compulsory Vaccination, 18 December 1882, pub. 1883, p. 4.
10 Collins, *Review of the Norwich Vaccination Inquiry*, p. 22.

18 The Great Pox

1 R. Blackmore, *A Treatise upon the Small Pox*, 1723, p. 206.
2 J. Burges, *An Account of the preparation and management necessary to inoculation*, 1744.
3 Sutton, *The Inoculator*, p. 58.
4 Simon, *English Sanitary Institutions*, p. 383.
5 Seaton, *Handbook*, p. 312
6 Farr, 21st Report of the Registrar General, 1861, p. 203.
7 J. Hutchinson, 'Report on two series of cases', *Transactions of the Royal Medical and Chirurgical Society*, 1871, p. 319. Hutchinson wrote a book on syphilis in which he quoted references to the series of cases mentioned in these reports, but got them wrong. They should be: *Transactions of the Royal Medical and Chirurgical Society*, liv, pp. 317–39 and *Transactions of the Royal Medical and Chirurgical Society*, 1873, pp. 189–202. I am grateful to Mrs J. C. Sen of the John Rylands University of Manchester University for her kind assistance in unravelling this problem.
8 G. S. Gibbs, *Vaccination Tract No.7*, p. 12.
9 12th Annual Report of the MO to the Privy Council, 1869 [c.208], xxx viii, p. 38.

19 A Genuine Conscientious Objection

1 Hansard (Commons), 19 June 1883. The motion, proposed by Taylor, was that 'in the opinion of this House it is inexpedient and inadvisable to enforce vaccination upon those who regard it as inadvisable and dangerous'. White records that when Taylor rose to speak the House was so poorly attended that it was nearly counted out, and that 'the great majority of those who subsequently voted against him were conspicuous by absence'. W. White, 'Sir Lyon Playfair taken to Pieces...', presented to the Third Anti-Vaccination Congress held at Berne, 1883, p. 1.
2 Parliamentary Papers: Report of an epidemic of smallpox in Sheffield by Dr Barry.
3 Royal Commission on Vaccination: Final Report 1896 [c.8270] xlvii, 889.
4 Royal Commission on Vaccination: Fifth Report 1892 [c.6666] xlvii, 547.
5 Royal Commission Final Report App. vii: 1897 [c.8613] xlvi, 1.
6 Royal Commission Final Report, p. 139.
7 Farr, 5th Report of the Registrar General [516], p. 215.

BIBLIOGRAPHY

Abraham, J. J., *Lettsom, his Life and Times*, 1933

Adams, J., *Observations on the morbid poisons*, 1795

Adams, J., *Answers to Objections against Cowpox*, 1805

Adams, J., *A Popular View of Vaccine Inoculation*, 1807

Al Rhazes, *A Treatise on the Small Pox and Measles* (trans. W. A. Greenhill), 1848

Alexander, J. T., *Catherine the Great*, Oxford, 1989

Annan, N., *Leslie Stephen: The Godless Victorian*, 1984

Ballard, E., *On Vaccination: its Value and Alleged Dangers*, 1865

Baron, J., *The Life of Edward Jenner* (2 vols), 1838

Baxby, D., 'The Natural History of Cowpox', *Bristol Medico-Chirurg. Journal*, 1952

Baxby, D., 'Is Cowpox Misnamed?', *British Medical Journal*, 1977

Baxby, D., 'The Origins of Vaccinia Virus', *Journal of Infectious Diseases*, 1977

Baxby, D., 'Edward Jenner, William Woodville and the Origins of Vaccinia Virus', *Journal of the History of Medicine*, April 1979

Baxby, D., *Jenner's Smallpox Vaccine: the Riddle of Vaccinia Virus and its Origin*, 1981

Birch, J., *A Letter occasioned by many failures of cow-pox*, 1805

Birch, J., *Serious Reasons for uniformly opposing the Practice of Vaccination*, 1806

Birch, J., *Serious reasons against vaccination*, 1807

Blackmore, R., *A Treatise upon the Small-pox*, 1723

Blane, G., *A statement of facts tending to establish an estimate of the true value and present state of vaccination*, 1820

Boerhaave, H., *Aphorisms concerning the knowledge of diseases*, 1724

Bright, U., *An evil law unfairly enforced*, 1886

British Medical Journal, Jenner Memorial Number, 1896

Brockington, C. F., *Public Health in the 19th Century*, 1965

Brown, T. (of Musselburgh), *An Inquiry into the Antivariolous Power of Vaccination*, 1809

Burges, J., *An Account of the preparation and management necessary to inoculation*, 1744

Chandler, B., *An Essay towards an Investigation of the present successful and most general Method of Inoculation*, 1767

Charles, Sir John, 'John Simon', *Journal of the Royal Sanitary Institute*, 1951

Clarkson, L., *Death, Disease and Famine*, Dublin, 1945

Collins, W. J., *A Review of the Norwich Vaccination Inquiry*, read at the monthly conference of the London Society for the Abolition of Compulsory Vaccination, 18 December 1882, pub. 1883

Conybeare, J. J. (ed.), *Textbook of Medicine*, Edinburgh, 1945

Copeman, S. M., *Vaccination: its History and Pathology* (Milroy Lectures), 1898

Copeman, S. M., 'Vaccination', *Encyclopedia Britannica*, 11th edn, 1911

Creighton, C., *The Natural History of Cow Pox and Vaccinal Syphilis*, 1887

Creighton, C., *Jenner and Vaccination*, 1889

Creighton, C., *The History of Epidemics in Britain* (2 vols), 1965 (repr.)

Crookshank, E. M., *The History and Pathology of Vaccination* (2 vols), 1889

Crookshank, E. M., 'The prevention of Smallpox', *The Lancet*, 1894, v.ii

Crosse, J., *A History of the Variolous Epidemic which occurred in Norwich in the Year 1819*, 1820

Dimsdale, T., *The Present Method of Inoculating for the Small-pox*, 1767

Dimsdale, T., *Thoughts on General and Partial Inoculation*, 1776

Dimsdale, T., *Observations on the Introduction to the Plan of a Dispensary for a General Inoculation*, 1778

Dimsdale, T., *Tracts on Inoculation*, 1781

Dixon, C. W., *Smallpox*, 1962

Downie, A. W., 'Jenner's Cowpox Inoculation', *British Medical Journal*, 1951

Downie, A. W., 'John Haygarth of Chester and Inoculation against Smallpox', *Transactions of Liverpool Medical Institution*, 1964

Dunning, R., *Some Observations on Vaccination or the Inoculated Cow-pox*, 1800

Edinburgh Review, Pamphlets on Vaccination, 1806–1809

Edwards, E. J., *A Concise History of Small-pox and Vaccination in Europe*, 1902

Emerson, R. W., *Representative Men*, 1850

Eyler, J. M., *Victorian Social Medicine*, 1979

Farr, W., 'Note on the Present Epidemic of Smallpox', *The Lancet*, 28 November 1840

Farr, W., 'On the Registration Clauses of the Vaccination Bill', *The Lancet*, 8 June 1867

Finer, S. E., *The Life and Times of Sir Edwin Chadwick*, 1952

Fisher, B., *Edward Jenner 1749–1823*, 1991

Fisher, H. A. L., *A History of Europe*, 1936

Fosbrooke, T., 'Biographical Anecdotes of Dr Jenner', *Berkeley Manuscripts*, 1821

Fraser, S. M. F., 'Leicester and Smallpox', *Medical History*, 1980

Frewen, T., *The Practice and Theory of Inoculation*, 1749

Fry, D. P., *The Law Relating to Vaccination*, 1872

Gale, A. H., *Epidemic Diseases*, 1959

Gibbs, G. S., *The Evils of Vaccination with a Protest against its Legal Enforcement*, 1856

Gibbs, G. S., *How and How much the 'Disease of Diseases' is propagated by Vaccination*, 1877

Gibbs, G. S., *The Evils of Vaccination with a Protest against its Legal Enforcement*,

1887

Goldson, W., *Cases of Small-pox Subsequent to Vaccination*, 1804

Goodall, E. W., *A Short History of Epidemic Diseases*, 1934

Greenhow, E. H., *Papers Relating to the Sanitary State of the People of England*, 1858

Greenwood, M., *Epidemics and Crowd Diseases*, 1935

Gregory, G., *Lectures on eruptive fevers*, 1843

Grundy, I., *Lady Mary Wortley Montagu*, 1999

Guy, W. A., '250 years of small-pox in London', *Journal of the Statistical Society of London*, xlx, 1882

Halsband, R., 'New light on Lady Mary Wortley Montagu's contribution to inoculation', *Journal of the History of Medicine*, VIII, 1953

Halsband, R., *The Life of Lady Mary Wortley Montagu*, 1956

Harris, W., *De morbid acutis infantum*, 1689

Harris, W., *A treatise of the acute diseases of infants*, 1742

Haygarth, J., *An Inquiry how to prevent the Small-pox*, 1777

Haygarth, J., *Observations on the Population and Diseases of Chester* (Philosophical Transactions), 1774

Haygarth, J., *Observations on the Population and Diseases of Chester* (Philosophical Transactions), 1778

Haygarth, J., *A Letter to the Syndicks of Geneva*, 1792

Haygarth, J., *A Sketch of a plan to exterminate the casual small-pox*, 1793

Heberden, W., *A Treatise on the increase and decrease of different diseases*, 1801

Heberden, W., *An Epitome of Infantile Diseases*, 1805

Hirsch, A., *Handbook of geographical and historical pathology*, 1883

Hodgkinson, R. (ed.), *Public Health in the Victorian Age: the Origin of the National Health Service*, 1973

Holland, W., *Paupers and Pig Killers*, 1994

Holroyd, M., *Bernard Shaw: The Search for Love, 1856–1898*, 1988

Hopkins, D. R., *Princes and Peasants: Smallpox in History*, 1983

Houlton, R., *The Practice of Inoculation Justified*, 1767

Hughes, E., *North Country Life in the 18th Century*, 1952

Hutchinson, J., 'Report on two series of cases', *Transactions of the Royal Medical and Chirurgical Society*, 1871

Hutchinson, J., *Syphilis*, 1887

Hutchinson, J. R., *A Historical Note on the Prevention of Smallpox*, 1946–47

Jenner, E., *An Inquiry into the Cause and Effects of the Variolae Vaccinae*, 1798

Jenner, E., *The Origin of the Vaccine Inoculation*, 1801

Jenner, G., *The evidence at large as laid before the Committee of the House of Commons respecting Dr Jenner's discovery of Vaccine Inoculation, and the debate which followed*, 1805

'Journeyman Engineer, The' (Thomas Wright), *The Great Unwashed*, 1868 (reprinted 1970)

Jurin, J., *A Letter to the learned Dr Caleb Cotesworth F.R.S. ... containing a Comparison between the Danger of the Natural Small Pox and of that given by Inoculation* (Philosophical Transactions), 1722

Jurin, J., Advertisement (Philosophical Transactions), 1723 (repr. vol. 33, 1724/5)

Jurin, J., *An Account of the Success of Inoculating the Small Pox in Great Britain with a Comparison between the Miscarriage in the Practice and the Mortality of the Natural Small Pox*, 1724

Jurin, J., *An Account of the Success of Inoculating the Small Pox in Great Britain for the year 1724*, 1725

Lambert, Royston, *Sir John Simon, 1816–1904: and English Social Administration*, 1963

Lambert, R. J., 'A Victorian National Health Service: State Vaccination', *History Journal*, V, 1962

Langton, W., *An Address to the Public on the present Method of Inoculation*, 1767

Lefanu, W. R., *A Bio-Bibliography of Edward Jenner, 1749–1823*, 1951

Lettsom, I., *Observations on the Cow-pox*, 1801

Longmate, N., *The Workhouse*, 1974

Lucretius, *De Rerum Natura/ On the Nature of the Universe* (trans. Latham), 1951

Macaulay, T. B., *The History of England*, 5 vols, 1849–61

MacLeod, R. M., *Law, Medicine and Public Opinion: The Resistance to Compulsory Health Legislation 1870–1907*, 1967

Maddox, I., *A Sermon Preached at St. Andrews, Holborn*, 1752

Maitland, C., *An Account of Inoculating the Cowpox*, 1722

Malthus, T., *An Essay on the Principle of Population*, 1798, rev. edn 1830

March, E. L., and Irvine, L., *Index to the Reports of the Medical Officers of the Privy Council and the Local Government Board*, 1895

Marson, J., *On Small-pox and Vaccination*, 1852

Massey, E., *A sermon against the dangerous and sinful practice of inoculation preached at St Andrew's, Holborn*, 1733

Mead, R., *A Short Discourse concerning Pestilential Contagion*, 1729

Miller, G., *The Adoption of Inoculation*, 1957

Miller, G., 'Putting Lady Mary Wortley Montagu in her Place', *Bulletin of Medical History*, 1981

Miller, G., *Letters of Edward Jenner*, 1983

Monro, A., *On Inoculation in Scotland*, 1765

Monro, A., *Observations on the Different Kinds of Small-pox*, 1818

Montagu, Lady Mary Wortley, *Letters and Works*, 1861

Montagu, Lady Mary Wortley, *Essays and Poems* (ed. R. Halsband and I. Grundy), 1977

Moore, J., *A reply to the Anti-vaccinists*, 1806

Moore, J., *History of Small-pox and Inoculation*, 1815

Moore, J., *The History and Practice of Vaccination*, 1817

Moseley, B., *A Treatise on the Lues Bovilla, or Cow-pox*, 1805

Nettleton, T., *An Account of the Success of Inoculating the Small-pox*, 1722

Newman, T. W., *A Letter to Mr Pitman* (pamphlet reprinted from *The Co-operator*, July 1869)

Pearson, G., *An Inquiry concerning the History of the Cow-pox*, 1798

Pearson, G., *An Examination of the Report of the Committee of the House of Commons* on Vaccination, 1802

Percival, T., 'On the Disadvantages of Inoculating Children in Early Infancy', *Essays Medical and Experimental*, 2nd edn, 1772

Pitman, H., *Prison Thoughts on Vaccination*, 1877

Plumb, J. H., *The First Four Georges*, 1956

Porter, D. and Porter, R. (eds), 'The Politics of Prevention', in *Doctors, Politics and Society: Historical Essays*, 1993

Provincial Medical and Surgical Association, *Reports and Papers*, 1830–47

Pruen, T., *On the Mortality of the Small-pox in London*, 1806

Pruen, T., *A Comparative Sketch of the Effects of Variolation and Vaccination*, 1807

Pylarinus, J., *Nova et tuta variolas excitandi per transplantationem methodus…*, Venice, 1715 (reproduced in Philosophical Transactions, vol. 19, no. 347, 1716)

Quetél, C., *History of Syphilis* (trans. J. Braddock and B. Pike), 1990

Razzell, P., 'Edward Jenner: the History of a Medical Myth', *Medical History*, 1965, 9, pp. 216–29

Razzell, P., *Edward Jenner's Cowpox Vaccine*, 1977

Ring, J., *Treatise on the cow-pox*, 1801–03

Ring, J., *An answer to Mr Goldson proving that vaccination is a permanent security against the small pox*, 1804

Rolleston, J. D., 'The Smallpox Pandemic of 1870–74', *Proceedings of the Royal Society of Medicine 1933–34*, 27, 1

Rowley, W., *Cow-Pox Inoculation no security…*, 1806

Rumsey, H. W., *Essays on State Medicine*, 1856

Seaton, E., *A Handbook of Vaccination*, 1868

Seaton, E., 'Report on the Recent Epidemic of Small-pox in the United Kingdom in relation to Vaccination and the Vaccination Laws', *Annual Report to the Local Government Board [c.1318]*, 1875

Shaw, G. B., *The Doctor's Dilemma*, Preface, 1906

Simon, J., *Public Health Reports* (ed. E. Seaton), 1887

Simon, J., *English Sanitary Institutions*, 1890

Simpson, Sir J., *A Proposal to Stamp out Small-pox*, 1868

Sloane, H., *An Account of Inoculation* (Philosophical Transactions), 1756

Smith, F. B., *The People's Health 1830–1910*, 1979

Smith, J. R., *The Speckled Monster*, 1987

Sparham, L., *Reasons against the Practice of Inoculating the Small Pox*, 1722

Spencer, H., *Social Statics [sic]*, 1850

Squirrel, R. (John Jones), *On Cow-pox*, 1805

Sutton, D., *The Inoculator, or Suttonian System of Inoculation*, 1796

Sydenham, T., *The Entire Works Newly made into English from the Originals*, John Swan, 1742

Sydenham, T., *Works* (ed. Dewhurst), 1966

Tebb, W., *Sanitation not Vaccination*, 1881

Timoni, E., *Clausula excerpta, ex historia variola. quae per insitionem excitantur* (Philosophical Transactions), XXXVIII, 1734

Timonius, E., *An Account of the History of the Procuring the Small Pox by Incision or*

Inoculation: as it has for some time been practised at Constantinople, (Philosophical Transactions), 1714

Tokswig, E. S., *Swedenborg, Scientist and Mystic*, 1949

Tomalin, C., *Jane Austen, A Life*, 1997

Trevelyan, G. M., *English Social History*, 1942

Wagstaffe, W., *A letter to Dr Freind shewing the danger and uncertainty of inoculating the small pox*, 1722

Watson, W., *An Account of a Series of Experiments with a View to ascertaining the most successful Method of inoculating the Small Pox*, 1768

Webb, S. and B., *English Local Government: English Poor History: The Last Hundred Years*, vol. 1, 1929

Wharncliffe, J.A.S.W.M., Lord (ed.), *Letters and Works of Lady Mary Wortley Montagu with Introductory Anecdotes by Lady Louisa Stuart*, 1837

White, W., *Swedenborg: His Life and Times*, 1867

White, W., 'Sir Lyon Playfair taken to Pieces...', presented to the Third Anti-Vaccination Congress held at Berne, 1883

White, W., *The Story of a Great Delusion*, 1885

Wilkinson, C. J ., *James John Garth Wilkinson: a Memoir of his Life*, 1911

Wilkinson, J. J. G., *The Blood: How guarded by God, and how violated by Vaccination*, 1877

Wilkinson, J. J. G., *Vaccination as a Source of Small-pox*, 1884

Willan, R., *On vaccine inoculation*, 1806

Willan, R., 'An Inquiry into the Antiquity of Small-pox', in *Miscellaneous Works* (ed. Smith), 1821

Wilson, G., *The Hazards of Immunisation*, 1962

Woodville, W., *The History of the Inoculation of the Small-pox in Great Britain*, 1796

Woodville, W., *Reports on a Series of Inoculations for the Variolae Vaccinae or Cowpox*, 1799

Woodville, W., *Observations on the Cowpox*, 1800

World Health Organization, *Smallpox and its Eradication*, 1988

Legislation

Poor Law Amendment Act (4 and 5, Wm IV, c.57), 1834

An Act for registering Births, Deaths and Marriages in England (6 and 7, Wm IV, c.86) 1836

An Act to extend the Practice of Vaccination (3 and 4, Vict., c.29), 1840

An Act to amend an Act to extend the Practice of Vaccination (4 and 5, Vict., c.32), 1841

(Jarvis's) Act (11 and 12, Vict., c.43) 1848

An Act further to extend and make compulsory the Practice of Vaccination (16 and 17, Vict., c.100), 1853

An Act for vesting in the Privy Council certain powers for the protection of the public health (21 and 22, Vict., c.97, 1858

An Act to facilitate proceedings before Justices under the Acts relating to Vaccination (24 and 25, Vict., c.Lix), 1861

An Act to consolidate and amend the Laws relating to Vaccination (30 and 31,

Vict., c.84), 1867

An Act for constituting a Local Government Board (34 and 35, Vict., c.70), 1871

An Act to amend the Law relating to the registration of Births and Deaths in England (37 and 38, Vict., c.88), 1874

An Act to Amend the Law with respect to Vaccination (61 and 62, Vict., c.49), 1898

National Health Insurance Act (9 and 10, George VI c.81), 1946

Parliamentary Papers

Report of the Royal College of Physicians on Vaccination, 1807

Report of the Poor Law Commissioners, 1840

The General Orders of the Poor Law Commissioners

Official Circulars of Public Documents and Information directed by the Poor Law Commissioners to be printed chiefly for the use of Boards of Guardians and their Officers, vols. I–VI

Report on the state of small-pox and vaccination in England and Wales and other countries, with tables and appendices, presented to the Epidemiological Society by the Small-pox and Vaccination Committee, 1852–53 (434.) CI. 75

Memorial presented to the President of the Board of Health, by the Epidemiological Society, on a proper State provision for the prevention of small-pox and the extension of vaccination, 1854–55 (88), xlv, 629

Papers relating to the history and practice of vaccination, prepared by the Medical Officer of the General Board of Health ('Vaccination Papers'), 1856

Gibbs, J., Esq., letter (dated 30th June 1855) to the President of the Board of Health entitled 'Compulsory Vaccination briefly considered in its Scientific, Religious and Political Aspects', 1856

Return of unions or single parishes in England and Wales of which the guardians or overseers have taken measures to enforce obedience to the Vaccination Acts, 1864

Copy of the Memorial on the subject of Vaccination presented to the Lord President of the Privy Council on the 5th of March 1867 signed by C. T. Pearce et al.

Reports of the MO of the Committee of Council on the state of the public health, 1859–71

Return for England and Wales, Scotland and Ireland, of the number of convictions under 'The Vaccination Act, 1867', 1868–71

Return of the number of vaccinations by the public vaccinators in every parish and union within the metropolitan district, as compared with the number of registered births, for 1869–70, 1871

Report and Minutes of evidence of the Select Committee on the operation of the Vaccination Acts 1867, 1871

Report from the Select Committee on the Vaccination Act (1867), together with the Proceedings of the Committee, Minutes of Evidence, Appendix and Index, 1871

Report and Minutes of Evidence of the Select Committee of the House of Commons on the operation of the Vaccination Acts (1867), 1871 (246) xiii

Return of the number of prosecutions in England and Wales 1870–75, under 'The Vaccination Act 1867', 1875

Vaccination Acts – returns showing the number of Persons who have been Imprisoned or Fined for non-compliance with the provisions of the Act relating to the Vaccination of Children; distinguishing Imprisonment and Fines; the length of Imprisonment undergone by such persons; the number of times any person has been Imprisoned being more than once; and the number and amount of Fines paid by any person who has been Fined more than once for the above-mentioned offence. 1st January 1870–1st January 1875.

Papers relative to the prosecution of defaulters under the Vaccination Acts by the guardians of the Keighley Union and a statement showing the results of the voting thereon, 1876

Vaccination Prosecutions – Copy of a Letter addressed by the Local Government Board to the Guardians of the Evesham Union... relative to the powers of the Guardians in relation to repeated Prosecutions against persons who have been more than once fined for refusing to have their Children Vaccinated, 1876

Vaccination – Copy of Report to the Local Government Board by Mr J Netten Radcliffe, on certain Cases of Erysipelas following upon Vaccination, in the Misterton District of the Gainsborough Union, Lincolnshire, and in adjoining Districts of the same Union, 1877 (433), xxvlll, 553

Reports of the Registrar General, 1839–79

Reports of the MO of the Privy Council and the Local Government Board 1873–78/79

Return of the number of prosecutions in England and Wales during 1875–78, under the Vaccination Act, 1867, distinguishing persons summoned under Section 29, and under Section 31; stating also the amount of penalty inflicted on conviction &c., 1880

Return showing the number of persons who have been imprisoned or fined for non-compliance with the Act relating to the vaccination of children; distinguishing imprisonments and fines, the length of imprisonment, the number of convictions more than once, &c., 1880

Report to the President of the Local Government Board by inspectors appointed to inquire into certain deaths and injuries alleged to have been caused by vaccination at Norwich, 1882 (385) viii, 613

Memorandum by the MO of the Local Government Board on the probable origin of erysipelas at the Norwich public vaccination station in June 1882; 1882 (395), lvii, 649

Reports of the MO to the Local Government Board 1879–89

Report on an epidemic of small-pox at Sheffield during 1887–88 by Dr Barry, with an introduction by the MO of the Local Government Board; 1889 (328) [c.5645] lxv, 45

Return of Convictions under the Vaccination Acts, distinguishing imprisonments from fines, and the length of imprisonment; showing also the repeated convictions and amount of repeated fines since 31st July 1889, 1890

Report of the Royal Commission on Vaccination, 1896
Medical reports to the Local Government Board 1889–99

INDEX